Unassisted Homebirth

Unassisted Homebirth

An Act of Love

Lynn M. Griesemer

Foreword by
Marilyn A. Moran

Terra Publishing
Fairfax, Virginia

Unassisted Homebirth: An Act of Love.

Published by:

Terra Publishing
4103 Plaza Lane
Fairfax, VA 22033-3019

www.unassistedhomebirth.com

Cataloging-in-Publication Data
Griesemer, Lynn M.
  Unassisted Homebirth: An Act of Love / Lynn M. Griesemer
      p. cm.
  Includes bibliographical references and index.
  ISBN 978-0-9661066-0-2
  1. Natural Childbirth I. Title
  618.4'5   97-91220

Printed in the United States of America.

This book is printed on acid-free paper.

Dedication

To the loving memory of Marilyn Moran who died peacefully on June 13, 1998—one week before this book was printed. Marilyn was an inspiration to me and was committed to sharing her birth wisdom for over twenty-five years.

To every couple approaching the love act of birth: may you find the faith, wisdom and courage to birth your baby alone.

Acknowledgments

to my husband Bob, who I am more deeply in love with as each day passes.

to all of my children: Robby, Melanie, Hilary, Christina and Millicent, who have helped me see and experience the world in a whole new way.

to Nicole Lavallee, for showing me the alternatives I had been searching for.

to my friends and relatives, who were kind enough to simply listen to my excitement and passion for this project. A special thanks to my new "birth" friends: Laura Kaplan Shanley, Valarie Nordstrom, Marilyn Moran (may she rest in peace) and Martha Pugacz.

to my father-in-law, Bob Griesemer, Sr., for his editorial wizardry.

to those who sent me their stories and encouraged me to continue.

DISCLAIMER

This book is designed to provide information about the subject matter covered. It is sold with the understanding that the publisher and author are not engaged in rendering psychological and medical advice or services. If expert assistance is desired or required, the services of a competent professional should be sought.

It is not the purpose of this book to reprint all the information that is otherwise available regarding pregnancy and childbirth, but to supplement other texts. For more information, see the many resources in the bibliography.

Childbirth is a serious event and should not be taken lightly. Couples who consider the unassisted homebirth option should understand the responsibility involved and always place safety of the mother and baby above all else.

The purpose of this book is to inform, share and encourage. The publisher and author shall have neither liability nor responsibility to any person or entity with respect to any loss or damage caused or alleged to be caused directly or indirectly by the information contained in this book.

If you have attempted to fit whatever mold and failed to do so, you are probably lucky. You may be an exile of some sort, but you have sheltered your soul. There is an odd phenomenon that happens when one keeps trying to fit and fails. Even though the outcast is driven away, she is at the same time driven right into the arms of her psychic and true kin, whether these be a course of study, an art form, or a group of people. It is worse to stay where one does not belong at all than to wander about lost for a while and looking for the psychic and soulful kinship one requires. It is never a mistake to search for what one requires. Never.

—Clarissa Pinkola Estes

Contents

Educators\Mentors\Advocacy

PART VI—Birth Stories

FOREWORD

In *Unassisted Homebirth: An Act of Love,* Lynn M. Griesemer describes the way childbirth will be commonly experienced in the new millennium, which is only weeks away, really. All other books about birth (with the exception of a couple by me) are as obsolete as a manual typewriter in a newspaper office.

Like many of us before her, Lynn gradually became disenchanted with the way her hospital deliveries had been managed. Her first four births were not bad in comparison to the horror stories some women can tell. However, she sensed that "something was missing," as she put it. So, after much study and careful consideration, she gave birth at home to her youngest child, Millicent, with just her husband, Bob, sharing the event. As you will see as you read this book, her intuition was correct! She missed out on something extremely important, and so did Bob.

After Millicent's birth, Lynn was so certain about the wisdom of giving birth privately at home with her husband that when the baby was just a few months old she started to write this book. In it she explores the myths of childbirth, how an unassisted homebirth unifies a marriage, and the secrets your doctor will never tell you. I could have used a book like this when I was expecting our youngest child. It would have made arriving at my decision to have a do-it-yourself homebirth with my husband much easier.

A valuable feature of the book are the responses of homebirth couples who filled out questionnaires, that Lynn had sent to them, about their private birth experiences. Especially significant are what the husbands wrote. Their words underscore Lynn's statements about the importance of one's husband personally sharing the event instead of his settling for what she called the "insulting" role assigned him during hospital deliveries.

Troy said, "It was the most wonderful, fantastic, marvelous experience of my life, getting to deliver my own baby."

Matt wrote, "Wendy just had to push once and Abigail slid out onto my left arm as I brought my right hand up to cradle her lithe body. I felt the electricity of life course through me straight into my soul."

Rick agreed, saying, "When I saw Timothy's head crown, I felt a bolt of electrical excitement go right up my spine. A moment later, I caught our son. I saw my wife give a big smile; her face was radiating with pleasure."

That radiant pleasure accompanies the genital expression of birth when it is experienced by husband and wife in a suitable environment, such as the dimly-lit seclusion of the bedroom.

Unassisted Homebirth: An Act of Love contains a brief, but important section on "The Childbirth Scam." One usually thinks of con artists as cheating ladies in their 80's. A significant portion of them, it turns out, specialize in preying on 'honeys' in their 20's. In order to enhance personal gain, they deliberately betray their responsibility to inform pregnant women in their care of <u>all</u> their childbirth choices.

My mother used to say about men, "You can't believe the Lord's Prayer out of their mouths." This seems to be especially so for those men who usually wear a white coat with a stethoscope around their neck.

Bookstore owners can start right now clearing the old birth books off their shelves because there will be no call for them once people learn about the existence of this thorough, inspiring, well-written exposé by Lynn Griesemer, *Unassisted Homebirth: An Act of Love.*

Marilyn A. Moran
Author of *Birth and the Dialogue of Love*
and *Pleasurable Husband / Wife Childbirth*

PREFACE

My first four babies were delivered by obstetricians in the hospital because I did not realize that I had any other <u>choice</u>. After four unmedicated vaginal deliveries, my husband and I chose to give birth at home, with no one else present. We were disappointed at the lack of information as we contemplated a birth without medical assistance (or <u>intrusions,</u> as we saw it). We discovered only a few unassisted birth resources.

Too many of us depend upon "experts" to provide us with information. Most of the data on pregnancy and birth assumes hospital deliveries. Homebirth literature predominantly supports midwife-assisted delivery. The ideas offered here are a combination of personal experience, theory and research.

Birthing a child is a natural part of life. It seems radical that babies are born in the presence of technology at the hands of experts, according to a calendar or clock. It is peculiar to give birth under formal conditions. Yet millions of women do just that. role of a doula too

The purpose of this book is to <u>inform</u> and <u>encourage</u>. I want to encourage you to move beyond your fears so that you can make new choices which will bring greater satisfaction to your life. <u>Our bodies are capable</u> of birthing unassisted. Almost any couple can acquire the knowledge and develop the courage to have their baby at home alone. We choose our place of birth and who will be there. What will you choose?

PART I

What, Why, Who and How

1

Introduction

You conceived your child out of love; why not bear your child the same way? If we let birth happen in the privacy of our homes, there would be an increase of marital closeness, personal confidence, mother and baby bonding, and family attachment. Birth outside the home and in the presence of non-intimate people interferes with these elements.

Birth is much more than a medical procedure. It is an act of love. Having a baby is a simple act of nature, yet so miraculous. Everything is designed to work smoothly, if only we would not tamper with it. It is silly to think that we can replace a perfectly designed process with an artificial system. Technology alone does not make for successful births and birthing babies outside the family unit, without regard to psychological, social, or spiritual considerations leaves a void in the lives of many men and women.

At some point during our lives, everyone will think about birth. Many of us wonder about our own births or the births of our parents; and most people think about whether they would like to have a baby and what to do about avoiding or achieving pregnancy. Everyone knows of someone who has a baby, whether it is a relative or friend. What we think and

> Men are alike, for they share the human situation and its inherent existential dichotomies; they are unique in the specific way they solve their human problem. —Erich Fromm

feel about birth is a reflection of our personalities and values. How we birth is a reflection of our faith and confidence and how we approach birth reflects how we approach life. Birth marks the beginning of parenthood and is central to womanhood, personhood, couplehood.

Bearing a child makes a strong impact on a woman's sense of femininity. Her birth experience will remain with her for a lifetime. Memory of her birth event can be summoned to conscious thought within seconds. Few other experiences in life can be remembered so easily and vividly.

A father is profoundly influenced by childbirth. Birth is especially meaningful when he accepts responsibility for an event which has been in everyone's domain but his for over a century. There is no greater joy for a father to be the first to see, touch and hold his own child. He will instantly know that no doctor, midwife or other person should be the one to accept this new miracle in their hands.

Our decisions and actions about birth are based on cultural methods. We submit to established procedures, often neglecting to question convention. The many reasons for birthing at home are presented in this book. When you question why something is done, you are questioning its usefulness. If your answer leads you to an unpopular solution or direction that you did not expect, you will have to decide what action to take.

One of the problems in our culture is that we do not like the act of birth. We avoid it. We fear it. We endure it. The secret to a satisfying birth is to embrace it, not escape from it. If we prepare for birth spiritually, mentally and physically and then welcome birth as a beautiful event, childbirth becomes a whole new opportunity for joy.

Who is this book for?

This book is for anyone who has ever had a nagging suspicion that something is wrong with doctor-managed birth. It also explores why midwife-attended homebirth is not necessarily a preferred alternative. This book is for anyone who is currently pregnant or intends to be pregnant in her life-time and is written for couples who will become parents for the first, second or third time. It can serve as a guide for those who would never consider an unassisted homebirth (birthing without an obstetrician or midwife) but want to change how they think about birth. It also offers hope for anyone who is trying to recover from a disappointing birth. The seasoned birther, the aspiring birther, the skeptical, the curious, and anyone who is interested in pregnancy and childbirth may find something of value here.

Why choose unassisted homebirth?

Why would anyone desire unassisted homebirth when there is a "perfectly safe" environment—hospitals—for giving birth? How could a mother put herself and her child at risk when a modern hospital has all the technology and pro-fessionals to take care of them? Many argue that it is unsafe to birth a baby alone. Midwives who attend homebirths often doubt the safety of unassisted homebirths, declaring that couples are incompetent when it comes to bearing their own children.

Studies indicate that midwife-attended homebirth is safer than birth in the hospital. This is mainly due to the expect-ant mothers' physical and mental preparation. A greater percentage of babies have problems or die in the hospital than at home.

Unassisted homebirthers report higher birth satisfaction. It is very likely that they experience much less postpartum depression. The father's emotional attachment to the new-born, the couple's closeness, and the emotional and physical health of the new family unit all fare better when there are no hindrances at birth.

We cannot dispute the success of couples who birth their babies at home, alone. Any couple who has given birth in the most private and intimate of settings has almost never wanted to deliver subsequent babies in a hospital. There is no comparison between the medicalized procedure of delivering a baby and giving birth in a natural, peaceful setting.

delivering vs 'birthing'

What this book is about

power of language

This book will cover what is truly a beautiful way of birth, and at the same time will address some of the dissatisfactions and myths about birth. This is not a scientific how-to book. I do not wish to lecture about the anatomy and physiology of pregnancy and birth or replace midwifery and obstetrics. I am not medically trained in obstetrics, midwifery or childbirth and can only offer basic guidelines on how to prepare for an unassisted homebirth.

This book will be a presentation of unassisted homebirth as it relates to psychological growth and development of the couple, the woman and the man. This book will address the question *why?* Why do some people choose to have unassisted homebirths? Why should we aim for an unassisted homebirth? Why are so many people against unassisted homebirths? Why should we care about this issue anyway?

I will also address some *how* and *what* questions. How does unassisted homebirth compare with traditional hospital birth? How does an unassisted homebirth bring a couple closer together? How does it contribute towards psychological growth? How is unassisted childbirth a feminist issue? What is the role of midwives in the birth process? What are some of the things that have gone wrong during unassisted homebirths?

It is important that men be fully involved in the birth of their children. Men do not talk about birth as much as women. I have rarely seen men write about the emotional, psychological and spiritual elements of birth, yet I know that the birth of a child has a profound effect on men's lives. Disinterest and a passive role at birth is the beginning of apathy in fatherhood. Obstetricians and midwives who orchestrate the birth event actually serve as surrogate fathers. You will have an opportunity to read personal comments written by the fathers who responded to my questionnaire (see Appendix C). I devoted a full chapter to men and birth and was able to gather very candid opinions from the men whose wives wrote the birth stories in Part VI.

My goal is to touch upon various topics of birth in general and unassisted homebirth in particular. All of the birth stories are personal testimonies from births occurring after 1990. Some of the variation includes: babies born at 36 and 43 weeks gestation, waterbirth, Rh- mother, breech twins. Babies were born in the amniotic sac and with meconium. One baby had the privilege of being born in the same house where three previous generations were born. Stories were submitted from couples who had four unassisted births and from a couple whose first baby was a Do-it-Yourself (DIY) birth. Couples ranged in age from their early twenties to mid-forties. The eleven birth stories you will read about are from couples who live in ten different states and Canada.

How you can use this book — [handwritten: I plan to look at how I see birth as a future doula]

The concepts in this book are intended to be applied to birth in particular, but can be applied to life in general. Couples avoid unassisted homebirth for the same reasons that people avoid change in their lives: fear and conformity. Many people live their lives in a comfort zone, not risking change because they dislike or fear the unknown, or are afraid of ambiguity, failure, success, or even what others think. They miss an opportunity for improvement as they cling to familiarity. Just as expectant mothers fail to set goals for their birth event, many people fail to set goals in their lives, while still others are unaware that change could bring them more success and happiness in life. [handwritten: I don't like the use of the word 'fail' here]

Just as those who wish to increase their knowledge, set goals and take responsibility will encounter more success and satisfaction in their birth events and their lives, so, too, the amount of mental and physical effort you invest in your child's birth and your life is often proportional to the amount of satisfaction and success you attain.

Whether you choose to read the birth stories first or read the book in the order it is presented, I hope that you find this book interesting and helpful.

My wish for you

I want you to move beyond your fears, birth disappointments and need for approval. If you are considering an unassisted homebirth, please give it serious thought. If you have had an unassisted homebirth, it is vital that you serve as a mentor to others. Men and women at the top of *The Birth Pyramid* provide inspiration for others lower on the pyramid.

Even if you do not desire an unassisted homebirth, you still may be able to apply to your next birth some ideas presented here, after considering what you think about birth and why. But most of all, I want you to attain greater love in life, a stronger marriage, and more wisdom and faith.

We need to replace the business-like way of having babies with an intimate and natural approach to birth. Our attitude towards family size and childrearing is shaped by our experiences and practices of childbirth. Your birth experience will imprint itself upon your mind forever. Make your birth experience the beautiful act it was meant to be, so that you will live with the beautiful memory you are meant to have.

[handwritten annotation: victim? blamey? things are often out of our control]

Young couples deserve to have all the information available in order to make informed decisions about where and how they want to experience the genital expression at birth. Neither obstetricians nor midwives are telling them the whole story. So, it is up to us laywomen (and their spouses!) to give it a try. —Marilyn Moran

2

My Story

The Birth Of Millicent

August 3, 1996

Not a day goes by that I don't think about the birth of Millicent. There's something appealing, almost erotic about conceiving and bearing a child in the same place, with the same intimacy. No event in my life has come close to deepening my appreciation of my femininity, concern for all humanity and faith and trust in God than my unassisted homebirth. I have never felt such euphoria for such a long period of time. My story is not so different from what most women's birth stories would be if they desired a simple birth and allowed nature to prevail. Our society has made childbirth so complicated that it seems unusual to have such an easy, effortless birth.

For me, there are so many similarities between the wedding day and birth of a baby. An opportunity to solidify an incredible love takes place. Forces beyond comprehension led up to my husband's and my decision to marry. They were also at work on our wedding day, the public recognition of our committed love. The births of each of our five children were moments where the force of love was at an all-time high. The significant difference between our unassisted homebirth and the other births was that those same forces of love were able to unfold without interference or distraction.

When we received the sacrament of marriage, the priest asked us two important questions: "Will you accept children lovingly from God?" and "Will you promise to love each other all the days of your life?" After answering "yes," he then said, "Let no man divide what God has joined together." I did not realize on our wedding day that this phrase was perfectly suited for childbirth. During our fifth child's birth, no one was there to divide what was so beautifully joined together on July 6, 1985. We feel blessed that our daughter was born simply at 4:00 A.M., in the same loving manner in which she was conceived.

Why we chose an unassisted homebirth

The idea of a homebirth first occurred to me after we had been homeschooling our son Robby for a year. That was in 1994 when he was seven years old and our youngest was 1-1/2. I was becoming more family oriented and tired of our society's impersonal approach and desensitized attitude towards everything in life. We decided on a homebirth not because of a negative experience, but as people seeking more meaning in life and an ability to realize our potentials.

Our first four pregnancies and births consisted of prenatal care with obstetricians and births involving minimal medication to no medication at all. And our first four children were born within eight hours of arrival at the hospital. Sure, we were excited about having each child, but something was missing. I knew that there must be a better way and wanted to say good-bye to the electronic fetal monitor (EFM), intentional breaking of the "water bag," ice chips, nurses recommending drugs for discomfort, pitocin to speed up a delivery, the baby treated as hospital property, and strangers (health professionals) just doing their jobs.

Sometimes life seems to be a series of acts where we assume many different roles. I yearned for an authentic birth where I did not have to put on a socially acceptable performance. I knew that somehow there was a way to have an intimate birth.

I remember the time I was left alone in the birthing room for over an hour before my second child was born. I could hear several other heartbeats as the staff rotated from one woman to another. What an impersonal, socialist way of delivering babies, I thought. My husband abandoned me for a snack and I was calm, bored, and not in excruciating pain. When the doctor returned to perform an exam, he found that I was nine centimeters dilated, and with his call for a nurse, the birth room dramatics began.

All of my life, I've always been a dutiful patient, respecting the opinions of "experts" and trusting their decisions. After all, they knew more than I did, didn't they? The medical establishment considers your medical history, but does not take the time to understand your philosophies about taking medication and your approach to pain management. Although I considered myself an assertive, persistent person, I did not realize that I became submissive in the prenatal and birth process by conforming to it.

I make many decisions based on a combination of research and intuition. I am motivated by love, new adventures and personal growth. One of my main priorities in life is the family—our particular family and the family as the foundation of a strong society. My husband Bob and I take matters into our own hands if we see that organizations or individuals fail us due to mediocrity, insincerity or lack of customer service.

Preparation

Preparing for an unassisted homebirth meant that I needed to be scientifically and psychologically strong. The initial idea led me to research. The most helpful authors included Sheila Kitzinger, Marilyn Moran, Michel Odent and Rahima Baldwin. After reading *Birth and the Dialogue of Love*, Bob was convinced that an intimate husband and wife birth was what we needed to strive for. Talking with eight other women who had homebirths and reading twenty other sources helped me a great deal. I came across all types of information—medical information written by doctors, midwives and experienced homebirth "authorities." I read about water births and homebirth from "hippie," Buddhist and Christian viewpoints.

All of the material was fascinating and each touched me in various ways. I was never so informed about childbirth as I was with our fifth child! Preparing for an unassisted homebirth was like cramming for an exam—six months of intensive research and I still felt somewhat unprepared.

Bob and I decided during the eighth month that we did not want anyone else at our birth. I assumed that I would give birth during the middle of the night. If our birth happened during the day, I was going to let our four children under age nine decide if they wanted to witness the birth, by leaving the door open or unlocked. The birth occurred at 4:00 A.M. and I thought about waking our eight-year old son. My husband preferred no human or mechanical witnesses and it ended up being just the two of us. Although I would have treasured a videotape, photographs or cassette tape of the birth, I was pleased that nothing distracted us from our birth. Writing about the birth afterwards was a wonderful way to relive and record the event.

Preparing for my homebirth was a journey of increasing trust—trust in knowledge, ability, and faith. Educational preparedness and excellent prenatal habits will not ensure a successful homebirth, exclusively. A strong spiritual base or trust in God is essential to develop the tremendous strength it takes to pursue an unassisted homebirth.

The pregnancy

As with all of our other pregnancies, this one was desired and occurred within the second month of attempting to achieve pregnancy. Although we practice natural means of birth control and are familiar with my fertility cycles, I was surprised that I had two consecutive months of 45-50 day cycles, being used to 32-day cycles. One reason for such long cycles was that we took an extended vacation to a place with considerably higher altitudes. Recovering from the stress that goes along with a vacation, we discovered the pregnancy in January, when I was about seven weeks pregnant. I began seeking people with information on homebirths and was not successful, so I went to my OB/Gyn (Obstetrician/Gynecologist) at the end of February.

I told my doctor at our first meeting that I was looking into a homebirth and that it was probably more of a fantasy than a reality since I did not get very far in my 45 days of searching. I told him I would let him know if I was going to go through with a homebirth. His attitude was neutral, but I knew I would have to make a choice whether to continue with his services. No doctors or certified nurse midwives will offer prenatal care in this area to a woman who desires a homebirth. What a shame! I wondered why it had to be this way—what motivated them. It is probably a combination of greed, threat of malpractice, ignorance and insistence upon a medical model. They do not want anything to do with people who are not willing to play the game by their rules. These doctors offer a full range of services to women such as abortions, elective surgeries, five to ten types of contraception and infertility therapy. Surely they could offer women a few prenatal appointments if they were really concerned about women's health and reproductive choices.

On the same day of my appointment, I met Nicole at a homeschool meeting. Little did I know that she was to become a major force in our decision to have a DIY (Do-It-Yourself) homebirth. She passed on valuable information and just watched as we came to our own decisions, never once trying to persuade me of anything. Nicole mentioned that some couples have a baby on their own.

I immediately dismissed the idea of having a baby at home without a midwife.

We searched for a midwife to come to our home, but there was such a limited choice in our area. There were only three "lay" midwives, one of whom would be on vacation during my birth. Another midwife attended births, but lived two hours away. We met one midwife and realized that our goals were different from hers. While we sought an intimate birth with minimal requirements, she was bound by state regulations and seemed to be too controlling a personality for our liking. I felt uneasy paying her in advance, being subjected to a "risk analysis," and being evaluated on my ability to cope with stress in life. She was too intrusive and made me feel subservient. She wanted to conduct periodic classes, but we just wanted to do research on our own. I concluded that a midwife is just another level of interference and regimentation.

We spent the months of March and April resigning ourselves to a hospital birth. Our plan started out as a desire to reach the hospital within thirty minutes of delivery and leave eight hours after the birth. The time I wanted to spend in the hospital kept getting shorter. After more research and interviews with others who had homebirths, we realized that we could do this ourselves and that it was not a dangerous or foolish risk. I would never put my health or the baby's health in danger.

I decided to continue going to my prenatal appointments with my doctor and did not discuss my ideas or intentions to have an unassisted homebirth. He would not understand and I decided he might be necessary for a back-up as well as for prenatal care. I attended a total of six prenatal appointments. With each passing day, I came to believe that if anything went wrong, I would not trust my medically-minded, business-oriented doctor. All throughout the pregnancy I knew I was wasting my time and felt as if I was serving his needs by complying with his business practices. I did not fully appreciate my beautiful state of being because the joy of pregnancy was interrupted by an obstetrician running a business.

I had to orchestrate baby-sitting for the other kids and spent anywhere from forty-five minutes to two hours at an appointment. I was scolded by a nurse for having sugar in my urine, had to sign a waiver when I refused the AFP test, and was put on the defensive when I told them I "needed" only one ultrasound rather than the three they routinely administer. The ultrasound revealed that the placenta was where it was supposed to be and the baby was not breech.

Because I did not have a network of prenatal caregivers and I was not going to contract services from a midwife, my options were either to use a doctor or be totally on my own. Since I was not well educated about prenatal care and needed to learn a lot, I felt it was in my best interests, medically, to continue seeing my doctor. I do not regret my decision to continue seeing my doctor, but next time I will choose an informed, experienced friend for limited prenatal care.

During my sixth month of pregnancy, I felt very confident to birth my baby without medical help. I got to the point where I absolutely was not going to go to the hospital unless there were complications. Even then, I would not want my current doctor to respond to any emergency I might have had. The more I discovered about hospital births through people who actually worked there, the more tension, fear and distrust I developed, but the more I discovered about the birth process, the less fear I had.

We received our birth kit at the end of July and had time to get familiar with it when Nicole came over for a visit. There were more materials in the kit than we needed, like the surgical gloves and other sterile equipment. I wondered if Bob needed to wear gloves, but Bob and Nicole chuckled at my concern. Can I be faulted for being a product of the American birth culture?

Since the preparation for an unassisted homebirth required confidence and courage, we did not discuss our plan with too many friends, acquaintances or relatives. We did not need any added stress, pressure, or negative remarks. Most of all, we did not have the energy to educate others while we were educating ourselves.

Throughout my pregnancy, I swam regularly and walked a total of eight miles a week. My nutrition was satisfactory and I was very athletic. My blood pressure was 95/65 and I felt strong both mentally and physically. I simply tried to detach myself from negative or stress-inducing people in my life. Carl Jones' book, *Visualizations for an Easier Childbirth,* helped and as the weeks passed, my excitement mounted as I anticipated a joyful birth.

It was very appropriate that the baby was born during the 1996 Olympics, since throughout the pregnancy, I considered myself in intense training for a major event. As the culmination of these preparations neared, I knew that the birth would go smoothly. A desirable outcome had already occurred within my mind; I was just living through the process.

The birth of Millicent Maria

On Friday August 2, I went for an early morning swim. I lost my mucous plug at 9:00 A.M., spent the afternoon with good friends and went to sleep at 9:30 P.M. At 10:00 P.M. I rolled over to discover that my water had broken. Even though I had no contractions, I called Nicole who told me to call her if I needed her. Bob and I made preparations for about an hour, and while he lined the bed and floor with plastic, I boiled scissors, got my tape recorder ready, and took a shower.

Bob prepared a crock pot of warm water, turned the setting low and had ten washcloths nearby. During the birth, Bob applied warm washcloths on my perineum, which felt wonderful, but I later found out that he neglected to add olive oil. Brown bags containing towels, baby clothes and other items were in the corner of the bedroom. There was a time I was going to bake them in the oven to sterilize them, but I was too lazy and did not bother.

We fell asleep by 11:30 P.M. and I woke up at 1:45 A.M. Contractions were five minutes apart and we sort of waited around for an hour. We did not wake the children having decided we did not want them present for the birth. We had three friends who agreed to attend the birth if we needed them: Nicole, our OB nurse friend and a neighbor to watch the kids. Nicole was the only one who knew that my water had broken. I saw no reason to alert anyone else.

I realized that I had no videotape or pictures of the pregnancy after the fifth month, so I had Bob videotape me for a few seconds, but the birth would not be photographed or videotaped. I was going to capture the sounds on cassette tape, but Bob did not want anything to inhibit him or us. He was right. We had already experienced birth as a performance and this time it would be birth as a truly intimate moment.

why was this Bob's decision

Bob was reviewing *Emergency Childbirth*, especially the part about cutting the cord. He was very comfortable with everything else. We had to laugh when he read,

> In over 95 per cent of the cases of emergency childbirth, though the emergency attendant will be overwhelmed with gratitude and widely praised as a hero, he can smile within himself at the knowledge that his simple tasks could have been performed by any bright eight-year-old. (White 1989: 7)

Our son Robby was eight.

At 3:15 A.M. the contractions had gotten very strong and I turned on our relaxation tape, "Carmel by the Sea," for comfort. Our radio was tuned to a smooth jazz station and the lights were dim. I stood up and bent over slightly during contractions and it was great to have freedom of movement rather than being on my back, hooked up to monitors.

During our homebirth, we did not want to perform any internal exams to measure cervix dilation since we trusted the natural process to unfold on its own. As a parent, I believe that trusting and respecting your child to make good decisions begins at childbirth and even in utero. Mutual trust and respect between parent and child have been more successful for me than adopting an authoritarian approach. A unilateral approach and attitude about babies and children begins at birth in most hospitals or in situations where there are paid caregivers. Any paid attendant at a birth event is likely to exert some type of management in the birth process resulting in the attitude that "I, the expert, know what's better than mom and baby." This is unnecessary and detracts from the birth and initial mothering.

As I glanced at the red numbers on our digital clock, I saw that it was 3:35 A.M. The most comfortable position I could find was a kneeling supported position leaning against the bed. I cannot believe what a major difference there is between delivering a baby in a semi-supine position on a table and the position of freedom I was in. I vomited in a plastic container and knew I was in transition. Bob applied some warm wash-cloths to prevent tearing. I did not think he knew how close I was to having the baby, so I commanded, "Wash your hands!" He did and then I said, "When I feel like pushing, I'll say 'push'." While in the hospital, I think I stopped my-self from vomiting and having a bowel movement during the pushing stage. In the comforts of my own home, in the pres-ence of my beloved partner, I did not have to hold back any-thing. During all four of my hospital births I felt that I was part of a performance. My husband held back tears of joy at the birth of his own children because he was in a public set-ting.

As my right leg started quivering and my moans and groans got louder, I knew that the moment of birth was near. I refrained from pushing and allowed the baby to do the work since I was afraid of tearing. Her head came out in one motion, rotated, then her shoulders came next. I thought Bob was trying to pull her out at one point. Bob told me to push one more time and after I heard her first cry, I pushed the rest of her body out. I could really feel gravity's pull against the large baby unlike in the doctor-convenient-birth-position in the hospital. During two hospital births where the doc-tors did not pressure me to push, the babies slid out with one or two small pushes. The other two times I was told when to push as a result of the doctor examining my body's readi-ness (while disregarding the baby's readiness). During the latter two cases, I put forth a lot of effort without seeming to get anywhere. My advice on pushing: take your cues from the baby, not the attendant.

With our homebirth, I could feel the weight of the baby while she was still halfway in me. This was the first time I wanted to watch it happening, but could not because of my position. I asked what the baby's sex was and he later told me he had to check twice to be sure—"It's a girl!" The next few minutes were a blur to me, but Bob was very calm and methodical. Later, Bob told me he just knelt there holding his new baby in awe. He placed her on the bed beside me, suctioned her with a bulb syringe and gave her to me. After a minute or two I saw that she was cold and I said, "Turn the ceiling fan off." We had forgotten to put a blanket around her. I just wanted to hold her skin against mine and try to nurse.

Bob clamped and cut the cord 40 minutes later and then the placenta was delivered. One item that was helpful was the "placenta-catcher" that I made one month before the birth. I got the idea from Moran's book *Birth and the Dialogue of Love*. After an hour of clean up, Bob and I continued to feel so peaceful and Bob commented on what a scam it is that we hire OB/Gyns and have babies in hospitals. Bob tried to get back to sleep at 6:30 A.M. for an hour or two. I could not sleep and as the sun came up I was looking forward to introducing the rest of the family to our newborn. It was nice and quiet and the kids were amazed to see their new sister upon awakening in the morning. They knew I was going to have the baby within a week or two and did not expect to meet her so soon. *again Bob, What the heck*

During the last stages of labor, I had asked Bob if he should go get Robby, but Bob did not respond to me. I think I knew all along that Bob did not want anyone there. Robby woke up at 4:30 A.M. and saw me sitting at the end of the bed with the baby, but he was half asleep, needed a change of pajamas, and went back to his room. I was sitting on the bed holding our daughter with the cord still attached.

What a pleasure to drink and eat afterwards! I drank pineapple juice immediately following the birth. One or two hours later I had something to eat. While in the hospital, it was usually anywhere from four to eight hours later that the hospital tray would arrive. On one occasion, I was forgotten at breakfast. Finally, when breakfast arrived, I devoured it, and did the same thing with lunch, which arrived only thirty minutes later! The freedoms, comforts and silence of our own home were truly cherished during these special moments.

I had so much adrenaline that I ended up doing five loads of laundry, cleaned up part of our mess, and began calling family and friends after 8:30 A.M. Nicole came over at noon and checked me for tears. She noticed a slight tear, unworthy of any stitches and told me that my uterus was moving back into place nicely. She also examined the placenta for abnormalities and found it to be in good condition. Bob read that it should be stored in the refrigerator in case we needed to transport to the hospital; hospital personnel might want to look at it. We kept the placenta in the refrigerator for two or three days, mainly due to laziness. We buried it in the back yard and the placenta was not only healthy looking, but the grass where it was buried thrived. We saw a patch of green grass in our brown yard during the fall and winter months!

After a few days of quiet family time, we decided to take the baby to the pediatrician. I went to my OB/Gyn three days after the baby was born. We were both in good health, but then again, I knew that and did not really need a doctor to verify my assumptions. I was at a point in my life where I was beginning to break away from traditional medicine, but I still subjected myself to certain hassles inherent in that system.

Happy birthday

We named our daughter Millicent Maria. Millicent means strength and loyalty. Maria is named in honor of St. Maria Goretti. This saint's feast is celebrated on July 6, our wedding anniversary. Maria Goretti signifies forgiveness and purity among children. When we baptized our daughter, my father-in-law gave us something he had for over 40 years— a relic (small piece of bone) of St. Maria Goretti, complete with authentic paperwork.

With the birth of each child, I have always given a gift to the other children on the day the baby was born. This time, it was a great joy to actually have a birthday party at home on the day of the birth. While I was making cupcakes in the morning, a dirty pan or oven triggered the smoke alarm. Nicole said she would go over to the smoke alarm and start fanning it. After a minute had gone by and the loud beeps would not stop, I walked over to see her standing up on a chair fanning the doorbell device! I silently laughed to myself and felt so jubilant to have such nice friends and family to share the day with. We had the party at 7:00 P.M. that night. Millicent could not eat any of the cupcakes and we did not have a present for her, so it was an unusual kind of party.

While we were celebrating our daughter's birth, I was also rejoicing about the birth of many new things happening within me. As each child has entered my life, I feel as if my love has increased and ego has decreased. Millicent's birth tested my faith, fear and love. I have grown considerably from this experience—as a woman, wife, mother, child of God. As a woman, I have come to rejoice in my feminine power of birthing a child. Some women experience physical pleasure while many describe an emotional serenity at birth. An unassisted homebirth left me feeling confident, ready to take on new goals. A new sense of mastery has taken over my womanhood and personhood.

As a wife, I continue to grow in love with my partner as we share a beautiful life together. After sharing an unassisted homebirth, our trust, closeness and respect for each other reached a higher level. We only wonder what is in store for us next and know that our marital bond is impenetrable and secure. Although we know that we are not immune to marital disharmony in the future, we know that we will be strong enough to prevail during difficult times. In our relationship, our spirituality provides a foundation that gives us guidance, support and hope.

As a mother, I take my responsibilities of raising our children very seriously and diligently. As a child of God, I have come to realize His vastness and power. I am more open to God's influence in my life. The energy from our homebirth has created a sense of peace and bliss that continues to fuel my life.

I'm grateful that we realized the possibility of having a homebirth with our fifth child and encourage lovers everywhere to at least consider unassisted homebirths. Do your research. It's not as frightening, risky or as radical as you may think! It's wonderful and was one of the best experiences of our lives.

If two people love each other there can be no happy end to it. —Ernest Hemingway

3

The Beauty Of Birth

Giving birth, at its best, is something a mother does, not merely something which happens to her. (White 1989:7)

An art, a science, an act of love

Our culture has not yet acknowledged that birth has such lasting impressions on the woman, the man and their relationship. As a result, our way of giving birth in America fails to provide a woman with a deeply enriching birth experience. Part of the problem is that men and women believe the myths of birth (See chapter 6). Women do not believe that birth can be a gratifying experience. They have been conditioned to fear birth and expect excruciating pain. Thus, birth is painful. If you perceive that you are not in control and that the doctor will deliver the baby, you set yourself up for something which *happens* to you. "Just take the baby from me," is the attitude many people have right before consenting to a C-section.

Beautiful birth: full of beauty; pitiful birth: full of pit (pitocin)

When birth is treated as a science and not an art or act of love, many deviations take place, most of them not in the patient's best interest, but to benefit those administering the science. My friend, Lauren, an obstetrics nurse who works in a nearby hospital, assisted a certified nurse-midwife at a recent delivery. The midwife had over twenty years of experience and it was her first delivery where the patient kneeled down to deliver the baby. The midwife was amazed at the ease of giving birth in that position. When I asked Lauren if they might now encourage women to give birth in a position more comfortable for the patient, she said, "No. The staff would not want to give up their control and way of doing things." So much for doing what is most favorable for the patient.

The comfort of giving birth would be greatly improved if just a few modifications were made. More births would turn out well if mom was not hooked up to the EFM and restricted to a bed for delivery. Treating birth sensually, sexually, and naturally would result in greater satisfaction and desire to give birth.

Birth is personal, sexual, tranquil, often painful, sometimes pleasurable. It is cultural, historical, magical, mystical, emotional, powerful and stressful. Birthing women and new mothers often feel connected to women of past generations and experience a feeling of connection to future generations. It is very difficult in a hospital setting to fully experience sexual and miraculous elements of birth. The woman in labor is more apt to experience the stressful, medical and cultural elements of birth.

Women giving birth in a hospital are completely vulnerable, as are their mates. An unassisted homebirth allows a husband to show compassion for his wife. The true beauty of birth is realized when a couple does not let anyone interfere during a moment that should be reserved for just the two of them. Childbirth is very much a love encounter and should be treated as one.

Not many people care about the "beauty" of birth. We are more concerned with the safety of birth, almost to the exclusion of all other factors. Even though most people assume birth is safest in the hospital, under a doctor's care, studies show that birth at home is safer than in the hospital. When birth is thought of as an art, a new type of respect emerges for the birth process as well as the laboring woman.

The Birth Pyramid

Because the birth experience is largely dependent upon your mental attitude and state of mind, you have the power to control and manage what your birth experience will be. You can "think your way" to an easier birth. Pregnant or not, you already have images about the birth process and its accompanying personal experience. If you don't like the present images, you can change your attitudes and state of mind in order to redo the images into something you like.

The Birth Pyramid is a model that can be used to determine satisfaction. The closer you are to the top, the more likely you will have a satisfying birth event. You determine your position on the birth pyramid, but reaching the top of the pyramid is not a competitive process: anyone may rise to the top and those who do often bring others up with them. However, there is a large segment of the population that chooses to remain at the lower levels. Remember, what you get out of your birth event is directly related to what you put into it: the greater the effort, the greater the reward.

Highest point on the pyramid: low-tech birth, high level of knowledge, high confidence, positive expectations, assertiveness, optimal body-mind-spirit health connection, high responsibility. Willing to make changes, seek personal fulfillment, follow personal desires and intuition, belief that the individual is the final authority of her condition, low need for security, can accept uncertainty.

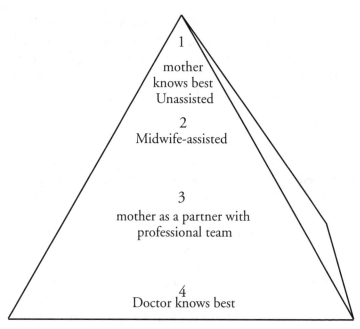

THE BIRTH PYRAMID

<u>Lowest point on the pyramid:</u> high-tech birth, low level of birth knowledge, low confidence, negative or low expectations, low responsibility, lack of full concern or involvement, dislike of change, high need for security and control. Goal is security rather than personal fulfillment. High concern for approval from others. Conforms to the system. Belief that the doctor, rather than the patient, knows more about the patient.

Level 1

The top level includes the small group of people who make a much greater effort preparing for childbirth than the general population. Their desires, beliefs and expectations are acted upon. They ask why certain birth practices are performed and try to find answers to questions others do not even ask. They know what steps to take and how to meet their goals. They realize that a healthy pregnancy means working extra hard; it is not a time to slack off just because waistlines expand. As their pregnancies come to an end, they become increasingly excited as fears diminish. They are never settled and keep on striving for optimum health of body, mind, and spirit. They embrace good nutrition, homebirth, natural birth and breastfeeding. Level one is the only position on the pyramid where the belief that "mother knows best" is dutifully followed. It is not easy, but the rewards are great. Those who attain this level are apt to be successful in other aspects of their lives.

Level 2

Those who are on level two are almost as determined as those at the top. They are not interested in unassisted homebirth, but they are very informed and determined about their pregnancies and births. They will be seeking a childbirth alternative, whether in a birthing center or at home with a midwife. They favor Bradley classes more than Lamaze or hospital-sponsored classes and are highly knowledgeable about birth. Their health is better than average and they tend to be more persistent and goal-oriented than those at lower levels.

Level 3

Those people who are comfortable conforming can be found at level three. Mediocrity is acceptable. All of their knowledge gained about pregnancy is through their caregivers. They might read a few popular childbirth books, but they generally rely on doctor directives. They will give birth in the hospital and probably take a hospital-sponsored birth class. Their social network consists mainly of other like-minded people in the same category. Whether they have a natural or drugged birth will depend on their ideas, fears, and intentions for childbirth. The degree of knowledge, responsibility, health-consciousness, persistence, and confidence they display will determine whether they are closer to level two or four. As they alleviate fears and strive for a lower-tech birth, they will rise to a higher position on *The Birth Pyramid*.

Level 4

Those on the fourth level seldom enjoy the experience of childbirth. They abdicate all responsibility to the doctor and are usually uninformed. They believe that technology will solve all of their problems and are more concerned with anything it takes to get the baby out and ending the pregnancy regardless of what is healthiest and most beneficial for the mother and child. They are the women you meet who suffer from all types of gestational health problems: nausea, diabetes, severe weight gain, toxemia. They have a hard time coping mentally and physically. They have practically thought and talked themselves into the notion that "pregnancy is an illness." Women on this level run the greatest risk of having a C-section. Since these women do not take much responsibility for their health or that of their babies, they are not likely to breastfeed and may have infants who are more apt to be ill. Oftentimes, their physical experience of pregnancy and birth is simply not as pleasurable as others.

Another group of women found on level four is those who have a strong desire to control events. Many affluent and highly educated women are found here. Women may be informed about pregnancy and birth and they often take responsibility for their pregnancies. Many do not fear birth and would not consider themselves conformists. However, their need for control and order overpowers everything else. They do not tolerate uncertainty. They will do everything to eliminate pain. Although level four consists of uneducated, fearful women who put all their trust in doctors, independent and ambitious women are likely to end up with C-sections and controlled birth experiences.

Why a "raw birth" is difficult

Many women have a hard time surrendering to a completely natural or raw birth because they prefer a life of order and control. Disruptions to this control are barely tolerable. While neatness, planning and maintaining order are important, flexibility and spontaneity are equally important.

Because girls are taught that maintaining appearance and control are primary values, an uninhibited birth is contrary to years of socialization.

Avoiding a raw birth is an act of cowardice. We are put on Earth so that we can contribute to our world as we prepare for our next life, and in order to do that, we need to grow in love, courage and wisdom. One way to gain courage is to face challenges. The purpose of giving birth not only perpetuates the human race, but gives women an opportunity to become more courageous. Welcoming a raw birth reveals strength—strength that is crucial for a meaningful life.

Birth is important to a woman's psyche

> A woman births with both her mind and her body, and psychological factors often determine how labor progresses. Birth is not an isolated event, but part of a continuum, an integral part of your psychological and sexual lives as a couple. (Baldwin 1986: 135)

A woman's sexual life encompasses her whole life. Crucial milestones occur when she menstruates and reaches menopause. Loss of virginity, birth of a child and breastfeeding are some of the choices most women will be confronted with. There are several challenges women may also face, such as hysterectomies, mastectomies, birth control methods, tubal ligations, infertility concerns, and any number of gynecological problems throughout their lifetime. In all of these situations, women do not generally talk with other women across the generations; they seek their doctor or women in their peer group.

Overall, society does not effectively deal with the sexual continuum, but seems to focus on one aspect of the whole continuum: sex. A vast majority of Americans focus on sex over any other element of the sexual continuum. Perhaps one reason we focus on sex is because it is the only part of the continuum which also brings great pleasure to men. Many people think that once a boy and girl emerge from puberty and become sexually active later in life, their sexual development is complete. People forget about the emotional aspect of sexual development, but instead concentrate on the biological development. The goal of sex is often self-serving as many go from one peak experience to another, chasing after more and more orgasms of greater intensity.

Most adults know all about sex and achieving or avoiding pregnancy as it suits their desires and plans, yet there is not a lot of knowledge about fertility cycles or having babies. What most people know about having babies is the negative impact it has on the self. "Birth is painful…. Babies keep you awake all night…. Children are a financial drain."

There have been many accounts of pleasurable birth, more often by women who give birth privately. That means outside the hospital, with only her spouse present, or in some cases, alone. Birth at home in the presence of midwives or other support people has also enabled women to give birth pleasurably. The reason for this is that birth is sexual and sensual and that a certain level of modesty is crucial for a pleasurable birth. Hospital births are more often described as tolerable rather than pleasurable. Expectant couples with very satisfying sex lives and love lives are at an advantage at the moment of their birth experience since there is a greater likelihood that their minds and bodies are mentally and physically strong.

Hospital deliveries take the couple's intimate moment and medicate it in a sterile institutional setting. The sterile environment of the hospital, the presence of strangers, or too many people detract from the emotional, sexual and spiritual elements of childbirth. The failure to integrate and express the complex components of our true selves results in alienation, desensitization and impersonalization. The typical birth experience in our culture does not lay a strong foundation for confident parenting.

The environment most conducive to the laboring body is that which supports the *inner event of labor*. —Carl Jones

Most women who give birth for the first time feel a greater sense of "womanhood." While I felt this to some extent, it was not until almost nine years later that I realized what was missing—intimacy, love, strengthening of the marital bond, increase in faith and confidence, expansion of my femininity and a chance for my husband to be an active participant and express his real emotions.

> Birth is a process of interplay between body and soul. It's a snapshot of a woman's state of being, a product of her personal history, her culture, her dreams, and her nightmares. It is an opportunity for healing past injuries and ripe with potential for inner growth, the kind that will nourish transformation into motherhood. (Armstrong 1990: 190)

The special connection between the mind and body are possible in an unassisted homebirth, but improbable in the hospital. The integration of the bodily act of birth with the psychological acceptance of parenthood begins immediately.

The power of silence

Blood, sweat, tears of joy and pain, saliva, mucous, vomit, urine, bowel movements. Almost every bodily release occurs during labor, resulting in the final adrenaline-packed moment of the birth release. Add to this scenario the emotions of love, anticipation, anxiety and stress. And you have a physically and emotionally intense event that can be best understood and appreciated only in silence. As a woman nears stage two of labor—the pushing phase—she is usually experiencing pain or at least massive pressure of the baby moving out into the world. In many instances, she does not

> Our entire life span is being medicalized.... Technological society dehumanizes people by encouraging a mechanical self-image—people viewing themselves as machines.... Capitalism adds that not only is the body a collection of parts; its parts become commodities.... Blood, milk and semen are for sale.
> —Ivan Illich

want to be bothered with a lot of noise, conversation or demands. The same is true in those few magical minutes right after the birth. Yet most deliveries occur in brightly lighted rooms, filled with people scurrying about their business, making mundane conversation. The baby is treated as an object to be examined rather than a person to be immediately loved.

Silence allows the body, brain and soul to replenish itself as it tries to recover from an altered state of consciousness. Silence, which is much easier to capture at home than in the hospital, allows fathers to contemplate their contribution and importance during birth and as a parent. Home allows you to transcend reality, while unfamiliar and anxiety-provoking people and places invade your silent space. Recovery time following the birth event varies for each person. Five minutes, twenty minutes, or a few hours of quiet time is critical for making the transition from pregnancy to parenthood, from a couple to a family. Any distractions or separations during this sensitive period can affect the early days as a new family unit, and jeopardize the chance for a successful rite of passage.

Experts have agreed that if left to nature, many births would occur in the early morning hours, when most people are asleep. This quiet time of the day is nature's way of providing silence for birth. Many babies are conveniently born during normal business hours. Some women make appointments for inductions or C-sections. Aidan Macfarlane points to a study of 601,222 spontaneous deliveries and noticed that there was a peak between 3:00 and 4:00 A. M., the time when a woman is likely to be in a peaceful emotional state, in quiet, comfortable surroundings. The onset of labor often begins during this time period.

Birth requires patience and trust. Patience and trust enter the lives of those who are open to it. Laboring women need time and space for concentration, which is best done in the absence of noise.

It was very liberating for me to give birth at home with only my husband. I have always known the importance of silence, but only recently figured out how to ensure silence at birth. At home I did not have to exert effort to achieve silence, but entering an altered state of consciousness during my hospital births required a lot of mental work. The only silence I had was based on my ability to retreat within myself. Meanwhile, I was not able to immediately focus on the new baby, which was in the hands of some nurse anyway.

Separation at birth

After the baby is born, it is often whisked away for measurements, shots and cleaning. My hospital births included separations that many others experience. After my first child was born, he was wrapped up and given to me within a few minutes. The nurse said she would take him away and be back in a few minutes. My husband followed her to the nursery where he took videos. I was left laying there, trying to recover from the episiotomy, making small talk with another nurse. One hour later, they returned. It was far too long and the baby was all wrapped up so nicely that I did not want to mess it up for fear of not being able to rewrap the blanket. I had not even looked to see that my baby was a boy, nor did I touch all of his skin. It was not until the next day that I did that.

With each child, I spent three days in the hospital, believing I needed a mini-vacation. Give the mom some rest before she goes home and has a lot of work to do, is what I thought. Also, during each hospitalization, I experienced a loneliness from my husband or the rest of the family, not to mention the baby, who spent a lot of time in the nursery. The nursery staff treats a baby as if it only needs or wants to breastfeed once every three or four hours. My fourth baby was given glucose water without my knowledge or approval. They could have simply brought me the baby and not confused her with an artificial nipple or pacifier.

After the birth of my second child, I was enjoying a peaceful visit with my parents and five-hour old baby. Interrupting the visit was the nursery room attendant who "needed" all the babies returned to the nursery during visiting hours! The hospital preferred to have the babies displayed for viewing rather than being exposed to germs from the many visitors. My parents had traveled two hours for a surprise visit and we stood there gazing at my beautiful newborn, separated from her by a glass window.

During each hospital stay, I let the nurses change diapers for three days. After our homebirth, I experienced meconium stained diapers for the first time. I thought this was abnormal because I had never seen it before. Thus, separation at birth can keep us ignorant and detached.

By submitting to authority, I took less responsibility and did not enjoy an immediate attachment with my new baby. On most occasions, I did not want to hold and touch the baby until I was told that everything was normal. Somehow I felt that the hospital was responsible for taking care of a disabled or "less than perfect" child. My love was conditional because of the setting I was in and attitudes I had, making me not very appreciative of the beauty of birth. I was just another new mother whose experience was limited by the emphasis on the science of birth.

It is customary for women to feel abandoned who have prenatal care and hospital deliveries with obstetricians. After almost forty weeks of appointments and classes, new parents are released from the hospital with little or no support. The mother may feel attached to her former caregivers, but neither side will have reason to see each other anymore. The business relationship has come to an end.

One of the most lovely aspects of our homebirth was that I was not separated from anyone—the baby, my husband or other children. We experienced birth as a normal part of life's continuum; there was no need to exit the home.

Giving up control

It seems as if everyone tries to control and manipulate events in their favor. When we fear something, want to avoid pain, want to escape from a situation or do not trust someone, we seek control.

Couples should thoroughly research what drugs the woman and unborn baby are taking rather than leaving it up to someone else. Some perceive that physical and emotional security are achieved by taking drugs. The pain may be more intense without drugs, but the ability to master that pain and influence the outcome is more likely during a drug-free birth; thus the expectant mother has more control. Those who choose to take drugs during childbirth are motivated by the avoidance of pain and are less concerned about those drugs passing to the child.

What may alleviate temporary pain is not necessarily the most healthy solution. Americans escape from the difficulties in life by using alcohol, illegal and legal drugs. The solution to life's minor discomforts includes *escaping and medicating*. People would be better off if they were to *embrace and meditate*. Healthier solutions are found as close to nature as possible.

> Wanting to control the danger and pain of the birth process, we invented medicalized management. It had unexpected and unfortunate side effects: It ended women's reign of decision-making in the birthplace and, in a Machiavellian turn, prevented women from experiencing the power of birth for herself. It also distorted the process of birth. (Armstrong 1990: 199)

The result is that women believe their bodies are untrustworthy and at fault when problems occur, so they submit to more medical management.

"Natural birth threatens mastery over self and environment." (Armstrong 1990: 217) Drug-free birth allows your body and the baby to be in control, whereas drugs provide an illusory, artificial experience. Birth and parenthood require an ability to adapt to change and uncertainty. This is contradictory to control. If more people agreed that being flexible is superior to being in control, women would come to the birthing room with different preparation and expectations. They would depart the birthing room having had a more enjoyable experience. Just as a loss of control during a peak sexual moment can bring physical contentment, the same is true for a birth which allows for a loss of control.

"The body-directed birth is gutsy and organic; it does not respect structure, linear planning, or bottom lines." (Armstrong 1990: 217). Because drugs make birth manageable, some doctors are uncomfortable when women labor and deliver naturally. Whoever is in control of the woman's body is in control of the birth event, so a drug-free birth allows the woman freedom and success. Women who take drugs during labor have to work harder to maintain control and power, but birthing in an animalistic, untamed manner represents self-reliance and self-sufficiency.

Two modern childbirth theories are concerned with control: one emphasizing nature and the other, intellect. Grantly Dick-Read suggested that birth pain is caused by fear which restricts blood circulation in the uterus and causes more pain. A woman who feels confident and relaxed during birth will experience less pain. The traditional Lamaze technique directs women to exert intellectual control to keep their minds off the pain. The goal is to be orderly and predictable, to be a dutiful patient. Lamaze encourages women to remain distant from labor in order to be in control. The Lamaze method assumes pain and teaches women to separate themselves from their misery. The Lamaze frame of mind is crucial for a hospital staff whose newborn care-giving function requires patient conformity and detachment.

The teachings of Robert Bradley and Carl Jones have been embraced more often by expectant women than obstetricians. The Bradley method teaches women to trust their bodies and informs women about many topics that obstetricians neglect. Carl Jones emphasizes visualization as a way to feel relaxed and empowered during birth. If you can maintain a positive attitude and high degree of confidence, your mind can practically control the birth.

It is difficult to feel control over your situation upon entering a hospital. Paperwork must be completed; rules and regulations must be followed. It becomes a battle for an individualized (as opposed to institutionalized) birth. A woman is put on the defensive to ensure she gets what she wants. Hospitals are brightly lighted, non-private, ungentle environments. Many women reason that they do not have to act tough (avoid drugs) for some idealistic notion (an unmedicated vaginal delivery).

Rather than trusting nature, women seek to control, manipulate and command it. A special birth requires the release of any inhibitions. Expectant women who acknowledge that there is a moment of intense vulnerability during childbirth can more easily resign themselves to the experience, allowing for growth and depth of their personhood.

Who should witness the birth?

Prenatal care, location of the birth, and use of pain medication are just a few issues couples must take into consideration. Another question is who to have at this important event. The couple may decide to have a labor coach, older children or other relatives present.

During hospital births, the deliverer of the baby will be there, along with one or two nurses. An anesthesiologist may be required by the hospital or insurance company. Oftentimes, the only familiar face is the doctor, who is usually the person who spends the least amount of time with the couple during their labor, delivery and post-delivery. The husband may be meeting the doctor for the first time in the delivery room.

Those who have unassisted homebirths have varied opinions about witnesses. Parties are sometimes organized during the event and other children observe or help. Very young children may be cared for by friends or relatives in another place. Some videotape or photograph the event. While who witnesses the birth is largely a matter of preference, a satisfying birth is largely dependent on who is at the birth. Where and with whom a woman delivers her baby will leave a lasting impression on her psyche, her life.

Top ten reasons to birth at home

1. You don't have to leave the nest to add to it.
2. You have more control over labor and birth.
3. Father can be intimately involved.
4. No strangers and unnecessary equipment.
5. Lack of interference—no one ridicules, hurries or coaxes you to take drugs. No internal exams or arbitrary demands.
6. Baby won't be treated as an object to be poked, weighed, measured or taken away for testing and experimentation.
7. Birth is safer at home than in the hospital.
8. Greater likelihood for physical and emotional pleasure; less pain.
9. Less postpartum depression.
10. Greater likelihood for a "peak experience"/self-actualization.

4

Unassisted Homebirth

Who, What and Why?

What is unassisted homebirth?

An unassisted homebirth experience is quite different from a birth experience in which a doctor or midwife presided. A married couple giving birth together will have to confront issues they would not ordinarily have to face if someone else was responsible for their birth. A certain amount of knowledge of the birth process is required. They will have to decide how they will deal with pain, fear and trust. A woman giving birth without her mate will have to completely trust herself and her abilities.

Unassisted means unaided by medical personnel. Medical personnel includes, but is not limited to obstetricians, midwives and someone whose livelihood is related to childbirth. They may have obtained their training formally, with certificates or degrees awarded, or more informally, where experience accounted for their learning. In most instances, medical personnel are bound by rules, laws and procedures, not allowing full flexibility during the birth process.

The couple, the woman alone, or in some cases, the laboring woman and a friend take full responsibility for the actual birth of the child. No one is hired to deliver the baby at a planned unassisted homebirth. No fees are paid or contract signed. There may be others at the birth helping in a nonmedical role, such as baby-sitting other children, meal preparation, or clean up. An unplanned unassisted homebirth is a more stressful and potentially dangerous birth where a hired attendant did not make it to the birth.

Homebirth is the process of having a baby in a place other than a hospital, institution or birthing center. In most cases, the birth takes place in the home, but the birth can occur in a cozy, comfortable place of the mother's or couple's choice. It can be on a boat or out in nature and is not necessarily restricted to the residence. The primary impetus driving couples toward a homebirth is the belief that birth is intended to occur in a haven of happiness and love. *The American Heritage Dictionary of the English Language* defines home as "the place where one was born or spent his early childhood, as a town, state, or country."

Unassisted, unattended, unhindered, husband / wife, couples birth, or Do-it-Yourself (DIY) homebirth refer to the same act. Jeannine Parvati Baker, founder of Hygieia College, "a mystery school in womancraft and lay midwifery," refers to DIY as "freebirth:"

> Freebirth is giving birth in fullest freedom without paying anyone to be paranoid for you. There are no costs at any level as what is valued is core responsibility, rather than buying someone else to take on this primal opportunity to cultivate responsibility. No doctor or midwife fees, no hospital and equipment bills and no cost to the psyche in endless cycles of blame for birth disappointments.... Freebirth is the movement from a smaller space to a larger one—one in which trust, not fear, is affirmed by the presence of lovers, rather than doctors / fixers. A couple feels more erotically in tune when they claim their privacy and much more likely to discover the "hands of God" without the hands of the experts involved. (Parvati Baker: "The Possible Family: Little House on the Edge of the Millennium" 1995)

The following are some examples of unassisted homebirths:

1. A couple planning a homebirth where they will be the only ones present call upon a friend to watch the other children. The mother received prenatal care from a midwife and did not make a financial agreement with the midwife to be present at the birth.

2. A couple, where one spouse is an obstetrician, gives birth in their home. No medication or technology was used. Several friends and family witnessed the birth. A friend who volunteered to serve as a labor coach was later given a monetary gift in appreciation.

3. A midwife who failed to answer her phone or pager does not show up for the birth even though there was a contract for her services.

The following are not unassisted homebirths:

1. The midwife arrives ten minutes before the birth and stands back to watch the father catch the baby.

2. A couple contracted services with a midwife who sits in another room during the birth just in case something goes wrong. She is still available for assistance and will most likely help immediately following the birth of the baby.

Who desires unassisted homebirth?

Most couples in America have their babies in the hospital, with an obstetrician as the main attendant. Therefore, homebirthers are in the minority and homebirthing is countercultural. This may elicit images of people who are anti-establishment or have a dislike or distrust of the prevalent medical system. Some people may assume that "hippies," farmers, illegal immigrants or lower income Americans without health insurance constitute a majority of homebirthers. This is not the case. Unassisted homebirth is a decision more often based on psychological factors than strictly financial reasons. Low income families could qualify for medicaid coverage for childbirth. Many homebirthers have health coverage.

People who desire an unassisted homebirth are often intelligent, well-informed people of various income levels, professions, jobs, religions and political beliefs. Those who have had bad hospital experiences and those who have had good hospital experiences may opt for an unassisted homebirth. In most cases, it is the woman's idea to have a DIY birth.

Many couples evolve towards an unassisted homebirth. The first child may have been born in a hospital attended by an OB/Gyn. The second baby may have been born at home with a midwife's guidance. Opting for an even more personal experience, a couple may conclude that an unassisted homebirth would be the most desirable way to have a baby. It is uncommon for first time parents to have an unassisted homebirth and those who have a DIY for their first child often have had some exposure to unassisted homebirth. Other couples intuitively know that an unassisted homebirth is how they want to birth their babies and may have had the idea before they met their partners or got pregnant.

The eleven stories which appear at the end of this book were written by mothers who are committed to their families in a full time capacity. Before having children, these mothers' careers and jobs included: photographer, secretarial jobs, registered nurse, psychiatric nursing assistant, veterinary assistant and purchasing agent. Education level varied from high school graduate to college graduate. Four of the mothers are either childbirth educators, doulas or studying to become midwives.

The fathers' educational levels ranged from high school graduate to college graduate. One father is a naturalist and director of a nonprofit organization while another is a postal worker and Coast Guard retiree. One is self-employed in the publishing business and one is self-employed in the roofing business. Other professions include a chiropractor, senior network engineer, logistics management, tool and die maker, electronic mechanic and Christian philanthropist. One father is in the Air Force.

The homebirthers profiled in this book were between 21 and 44 years of age at the time of their DIY birth. The babies were the firstborn through the seventh child. Some women have had previous C-sections or natural hospital births. Some describe their hospital, birthing center or home attended birth experiences as good, while others were not at all pleased with previous deliveries. The couples featured in this book are married, but single parents also choose DIYs. Some women have chosen to give birth alone or with the help of another friend or older child. The variation of birth stories mentioned in this book include: waterbirth, firstborn baby, breech twins, babies born at 36 and 43 weeks gestation, fourth generation baby born in the same house, and four DIYs born to the same couple.

Birth situations included Rh- blood, meconium, baby born in amniotic sac, cord wrapped around the neck, and shoulder dystocia. Others have had physical, emotional or marital problems shortly before or after the births. One couple had a DIY following four miscarriages. Another couple's baby died from a congenital heart malfunction two months following a DIY, and several years later they had another DIY. Those who choose DIY birth experience the same joys and struggles of life like anyone else.

Since many homebirthers are committed to childbearing and childrearing, it is not surprising to find that all of the mothers are breastfeeding proponents. Many families believe in the family bed and some nurse their babies for more than two years. Most of the families do not support the practice of circumcision or immunizations. Television is rare in many of these households and the families prefer to spend more time conversing with each other or reading together. Healthy eating habits, eating at least one meal together and daily prayer are a part of many family rituals. Some families do not practice any method of birth control, while others seek to avoid or achieve pregnancy utilizing the concepts of Natural Family Planning. Many families prefer homeopathic, herbal remedies, chiropractic and natural solutions to life's discomforts rather than seeking traditional medical care. However, a few families use traditional medicine, but not aggressive treatments. Many families use cloth diapers, while others prefer disposables. Some families do not leave their children with baby sitters and find they are criticized for engaging exclusively in family activities.

Homeschooling fits in with the desired lifestyle of many homebirthers. Parents are committed to raising their children with a solid foundation based on values passed from mature parents to children. When children spend a majority of time in a classroom setting with a teacher and young, immature children of the same age, the parents have less time to influence their own child's development.

Many families enjoy church activities, volunteering and other events where the children can interact with people of different ages. Traveling, sightseeing, visiting historic towns and museums, telling stories and reading together are some activities DIY families cherish. Also, walking, biking, basketball, and other sports are important to many of the families.

In addition to possessing the qualities mentioned at the top of *The Birth Pyramid*, most DIYers are less fearful, more assertive, and more self-reliant than others. They tap into their mental and spiritual reserves. They have definitely thought about birth, decided what they want and do not want in a birth experience and have pursued their goals.

People who desire unassisted homebirth often exhibit characteristics of what psychologist Abraham Maslow has described as "self-actualization."

> Self-actualized adults are relatively unfrightened by the unknown, the mysterious, the puzzling, and often positively attracted by it.... They do not cling to the familiar, nor is their quest for the truth a catastrophic need for certainty, safety, definiteness, and order.... They have less need of other people, are less afraid of them and less hostile against them. They do not fear their impulses, emotions or

thoughts. This approval and acceptance of their deeper selves makes it possible to perceive bravely the real nature of the world and allows them to be spontaneous.... They are ruled by the laws of their own character rather than by the rules of society. (Maslow 1968: 138-141)

Why someone would want an unassisted homebirth

Those who opt for an unassisted homebirth cite various reasons. It is not always done because a couple was unable to find an attendant to come to their home, nor is it done because they are opposed to hospitals. Unassisted homebirths are carried out because of some of the reasons outlined in the next several pages.

Women choose to deliver at home *because* the medical establishment has defined them as "high-risk." Judie and Peter were not satisfied with the quality of care from the midwives at a New Jersey birthing center. "Once they learned we were expecting twins," says Judie, "it seemed that the control over our pregnancy was given almost completely to the established medical procedures for having multiple births." The lack of respect for the couple's convictions was enough to make this couple seek another alternative.

According the Charles Colson,

People don't pick a vision (or make a decision) piecemeal, as they might pick a bouquet of flowers in a garden. They come to such convictions (or decisions) within the framework of a broader set of...assumptions and ideals—more like accepting a story, with all of its internal rules and consistencies. And just as beliefs are not selected one at a time (what might be called the salad-bar theory of decision-making), long held beliefs do not fall one at a time. In the absence of a deeper conversion of perspective...minds are rarely changed on single policy matters, no matter how persuasive our arguments. (Balizet 1996: 181)

Love

The main reason couples desire unassisted birth can be attributed to the universal need for love. Love is a human emotion that cuts across all international, economic, social, racial and religious boundaries. That is why we cannot stereotype homebirthers into any one group.

Love is a feeling which arises without conscious effort. Childbirth is a love act involving the triangle of man, woman and child, but people are unaware that it is an intimate occurrence. Those who have decided to have an unassisted homebirth do not want anything to interfere with the love act of childbirth.

The presence of a midwife interferes with the expression of love between the couple. Many couples who desire a DIY often have a deep love for each other that they could not think of having a child under any other circumstance. Many couples feel their love intensifying (especially leading up to and after a DIY birth). They wonder how it is even possible to grow more deeply in love.

Greater intimacy

Life has become so fast paced that people seem to rush from one activity to another, trying to outdo one another, seldom slowing down to appreciate the basic things in life. They end up exhausted, unable to excel in any one area. In *Childhood's Future* (1990), Richard Louv described modern life as a "programmed generation," where activities and family time are constantly structured. He believes that many family members do not adequately connect with each other, creating an intimacy void which contributes to the emotional neglect of children, and increased stress in the family. People crave love and a deeper connection to their mates and families. Perhaps a little more simplicity is needed.

Respect is what we owe; love, what we give. —Philip J. Bailey

Most people do not take the time to actively pursue increased levels of intimacy. Lack of enough intimacy in our lives manifests itself in subtle ways: weight gain, substance abuse, meaningless activities to fill time and other escapist behaviors. Unassisted childbirth among lovers is a beautiful way to reclaim the intimacy that is so desperately needed.

News stories and entertainment depicting violence and immorality are shown daily and cause a gradual desensitization of our reactions to abhorrent crime and the misfortunes of others. Some people even preoccupy themselves with the misfortunes of others so that energy is diverted away from forming intimate connections.

It is rare that entire families take more than fifteen minutes a day to converse with each other. How often do you see families set aside time to be with each other and not in any structured activity? American families struggle in their efforts to take regular vacations together or to establish their own traditions. The busyness of life has practically replaced intimacy and connectedness in many families.

Lovers can recapture intimacy by having their babies alone. An intimate family event is possible when older children witness the birth. What better way is there to teach others about sex and responsibility than to include them in a natural birth? Rick and Patricia Kohl of Hopkinton, NY gave their oldest daughter Regina various responsibilities during two DIY births. Regina was seventeen during the first DIY birth and an "old pro" at the next DIY birth four years later. While Regina's American contemporaries were engaging in casual sex, worrying about pregnancy and sexually transmitted diseases, Regina was witnessing the healthy benefits of sexuality and unselfish love.

Those who had a hospital birth before having an unassisted homebirth were looking, in part, for greater intimacy in the process of delivering their babies. In most cases, couples evolve towards an unassisted homebirth and do not suddenly discover a better way to have a baby. You will rarely see a couple have a baby at home and then desire a hospital birth with subsequent babies.

As I have gotten older, I have become more private and introspective, perhaps more eccentric, but at the same time outward-focused and concerned for others. A husband and wife homebirth fulfilled my yearning for modesty and privacy. No other type of birth could; birth with a doctor, midwife, or friend present would have interfered with the pursuit of intimacy.

Unassisted homebirth is not just about "place"

Perhaps the first choice a person makes about the birth is where it will take place. Proponents of midwifery argue that a woman *births* her baby at home and *delivers* her baby at a hospital, as if place was the only factor in helping to create a pleasurable birth experience. Birthing (or delivering) depends not on location of the birth, but how much responsibility, power and control the mother takes for the birth. A good birth occurs in a place where the mother is able to be mentally and physically relaxed. Her state of mind is more important than location. Certain people's presence may be more detrimental than the place where the baby will be born. Successful births are ones where the woman can look back on the event and feel a sense of triumph and confidence. Her expectations and goals were met.

View of birth as a natural process

Childbirth for the masses is a hurried, impersonal process. Upon entering the hospital, a woman is often "put on the clock," unbeknownst to her. If her labor is not progressing in accordance with the doctor's or staffs approval, drugs may be given to speed up labor. If the pain is too unbearable, she often requests more drugs. This may cause her to lose some physical sensation and control, resulting in more intervention to facilitate the process. Forceps and vacuum extractors are used to drag the baby out. Many C-sections are performed because of a "failure to progress."

And what about the woman who passes her "due date?" Induction has become more prevalent in recent times. Some women are induced not because of a severe health hazard, but because the estimated gestational date has passed. A woman's initial estimate of her due date may be inaccurate, the ultrasound reading may be in error up to fifteen days and other exams are not exact. Women who have gone past forty-two weeks gestation have delivered healthy babies without being induced. Others are induced as a result of a health problem that could have been controlled and they give birth to premature babies.

In addition to lacking love and intimacy, current childbirth practices do not respect the natural unfolding of events. If unborn babies could talk, they would be shouting in utero, "Please, everyone, just wait! I will not fail you. I will come out in my own time, not yours."

Doctors may say that birth is a natural process, but their actions, in general, reveal otherwise. Amniotomies, time limits imposed on women to deliver vaginally and the supported supine position of giving birth are common rituals. Pressure to receive pain relieving drugs and yanking out the placenta within ten minutes are standard practice.

Most people, however, respect the medical establishment and hold doctors in such high regard at the expense of their own confidence and knowledge. In a society that views childbirth as something to be managed or tampered with, you can see why a hospital, or unnatural setting is the preferred place of birth, causing the outcome to be something other than a "natural" experience.

Abdicating responsibility and letting the doctor take full control of pregnancy and childbirth leads to a mediocre birth experience. Perhaps one reason women do not want more children is because the pregnancy and birth experience is not a joyous one.

The acceptance that birth is a natural process enables greater freedoms for the laboring mother. She is free to eat, use herbs, drink tea, massage, move, walk and give birth in whatever position feels comfortable at the moment. She is free to interact with her lover in any way she pleases.

The father of the baby benefits from a natural birth. When birth is seen as a natural process and allowed to occur in the comfort of one's home without the presence of doctors or midwives, the father will be more inclined to surrender to his emotions and display his vulnerabilities. Birth, occurring outside a comfortable natural setting, pressures the male to exhibit a socially acceptable emotional state. With midwives and too many people in attendance, fathers subconsciously feel that babies are a woman's work, a spectator's event, and not a couple's sacred creation.

Belief that birth should not include separation

"What God has joined, let no man divide." After eleven years of marriage, it struck me that this wedding vow was also intended for childbirth. That phrase not only has significance for married couples to remain faithful and committed to each other, but can be applied to them as they expand their family unit. Every time an obstetrician, midwife or third party takes control or responsibility for the birth act away from the couple, the couple is being divided or separated. The father sits on the sidelines as a spectator, rather than in the forefront. The couple is robbed of a milestone crucial to their development as parents.

In traditional hospital childbirth, the husband is relegated to picture taker, breathing coach or errand runner. It is common to joke that the woman in labor is angry at the husband for "causing" such great pain. Anger rather than positive energy is directed towards him. Women are encouraged to form a bond with a labor coach, midwife or nurse rather than with their lovers. This emotional separation between the father and the birth creates a distance between the father and mother as well as the father and child.

The events following childbirth in the hospital are ones of separation and anxiety. The ritual of washing, weighing and measuring the baby takes precedence over giving the baby to the mother to touch, feel, hold and nurse.

Some couples decide that the woman will have the baby alone. These couples believe that the physical separation between the lovers during the birth is desirable or that the presence of the father is unnecessary. The woman is truly autonomous and independent with nobody separating her from the ability to experience tremendous growth in the areas of trust and confidence. Laura Kaplan Shanley described her experiences of birthing alone and addressed the issue of autonomy in *Unassisted Childbirth*. Twenty years later, she and her husband David are still very close.

When viewed as a natural event, it follows that childbirth should take place in comfortable surroundings, where there is no break in the natural flow of events. This is not possible when a couple has to pack to go to a hospital or birthing center. In fact, these settings attempt to mimic a cozy, home-like atmosphere, but when it comes to birth, "There's no place like home."

Leaving home to go have my fourth child in the hospital was so stressful that labor slowed dramatically. I thought that labor should progress rapidly since I was not in danger of delivering my child outside of the hospital. Three years later while preparing for our DIY birth, I came across a more logical explanation of why labor may slow down:

> When under stress our bodies produce catecholamines, or 'stress hormones,' the best-known of which are adrenaline and noradrenaline. This is normal and advantageous under most circumstances, because catecholamines help the body adjust to stress. If the stress is excessive, however, or goes on for too long, the body exhausts its resources and can no longer adjust to the stress. When catecholamine

---

Birth without violence breeds children who are strong, because they are free, without conflict. Free and fully awake.
—Frederick Leboyer

levels rise abnormally in a woman in labor, her uterus contractions become weaker or spasmodic, dilatation of the cervix is slower, and labor is longer. Sometimes the uterus
simply stops contracting for a while. This often occurs when
a woman first arrives in the hospital, even when contractions have been strong and regular at home. The rise in
catecholamine levels has the effect of making her more
anxious, which also means that she feels more pain. This
in turn further increases catecholamine levels. It is a vi-
cious circle. (Kitzinger 1991: 18)

People who choose to have unassisted homebirths may
have at least one child already. It is so wonderful to remain
at home and not separated from the family. The children
may get to participate in the event and experience the natural beauty of birth. The interruption of leaving the family
nest to add to it seems absurd.

Dissatisfaction

Childbirth alternatives are on the rise, as many women
become more selective about their doctors and place of birth.
Some search for a childbirth educator and labor coach. Disappointment is inevitable for the subservient patient who has
specific expectations and desires for her birth. Women who
use such phrases as "they *allowed* me" and "give me something
for pain," position themselves to become victims.

A previous bad experience gives the couple good reason
to ponder what they want in their next birth experience.
Perhaps a C-section was performed and the mother feels it
was not warranted. Or, a good physical experience overall,
but a void in the emotional experience leaves the mother
hoping and wishing for something different. Often, she does
not know the solution. In many cases she will return to the
hospital to have future babies, and in some cases, the couple
will contract with a midwife to deliver the baby in their home.

Many couples are very happy with a midwife-attended
homebirth. There are others who feel that they did not need
the midwife. As parental experience and confidence increase,

the couple may desire a DIY birth. Whether the birth occurred in the hospital or at home with other attendants, there may have been a realization that childbirth was phony, impersonal, or a performance. Dissatisfied that a private event was somehow public, the couple seeks a private affair for their next birth.

Questionnaire results

When asked to state why they had a DIY birth, couples reported the following:

> * I believe that homebirth is the safest and most rewarding way to give birth. We were exceptionally educated and prepared for it. I'm a fast birther, so the distance to the hospital is a factor. I was dissatisfied with local choices and cost. I did not want to feel like I was "performing."

> * It was so important for us to be relaxed and comfortable during this high point in our lives together, a joyous occasion as God intended. Medical intervention has always caused great fear and tension in me. We believe that this type of birth is the absolute best start for our babies.

> * I longed to have a birth as I believed God wanted it: quiet, peaceful and natural. My C-section was unnecessary and my other two hospital births were full of poking, prodding and pitocin. Hospitals seem a very unusual place for childbirth.

> * Why not? The only sensible place to have a birth is at home since birth is a natural, simple gravity process, where the Creators get it out and we got it there in the first place. No strange men should be between a woman's legs at a holy process no matter what the title or degree.

* I read Marilyn Moran's book *Birth and the Dialogue of Love*, and it made good sense. I was confident we could do it and proved it could be done alone, since I started childbirth with a C-section.

* I have a strong commitment to homebirth. I am unwilling to bend to the rules of "the system," many of which are arbitrary. I have a desire for a deeper spiritual, emotional experience.

Why someone might not want a homebirth

Because birth is viewed as extremely painful, dangerous, and something to be feared, most people do not embrace the idea of a birth at home, never mind an unattended birth. The misconception that childbirth is the culmination of an illness (pregnancy) leads women to believe they need drugs. Homebirthers cannot resort to pain medication. Visualizations, meditation, prayer, positive affirmations and a positive attitude replace the use of drugs.

Those who want to control every aspect of life prefer to use drugs to manage pain and the unknown. Hospitals are a place to go when you are ill or have an emergency. Pain accompanies medical emergencies. The perception that birth is painful and risky goes uncorrected by a staff who exists to fulfill institutional goals. Doctors will take all of the burdens of childbirth away. Pregnant mothers who are willing to go along with a drugged birth cannot understand how or why someone could experience an unmedicated birth. Those who think the hospital is a much safer and comfortable environment will never entertain the idea of a homebirth.

Giving birth at home requires a high level of self-discipline, trust and confidence. A couple who lacks any of those qualities has forty weeks to prepare. Some women are uninterested, unwilling or unable to ensure a healthy pregnancy. Many men are complacent or view childbirth as women's work, something outside the realm of their responsibility or participation.

Sadly, many marriages are not strong enough to endure an unassisted homebirth. If an unassisted homebirth is going to pose incredible stress on the couple, they will not be able to cope with the general responsibilities or any problems that may arise during the birth. An intimate birth requires compassion and trust. A troubled marriage might be better off birthing in a place with medical or personal support.

Women who have had bad previous experiences may be reluctant to have an unassisted homebirth. Each individual must make a decision based on whether he or she would feel safe and comfortable. Many will tell you that if you are a teen, in your forties, have had at least five children, bear a child before 38 weeks or after 42 weeks gestation, have a breech presentation, have anemia or gestational diabetes, have Rh negative blood, or are obese you are considered high-risk and should seek medical attention. I have known women to give birth unassisted in all of those categories. The families are convinced that the mother and child enjoyed better health and a more dignified birth than if they had been in a hospital, under a doctor's care. As long as the couple is knowledgeable and calm, they often do fine in what others label as high-risk.

Who should not have a homebirth?

Couples should do their own assessment based on the current pregnancy and by considering previous pregnancies and births. If they decide that they are in a high-risk category, they should remember that a safe, healthy delivery should be the goal of all pregnancies.

Most pregnancies end in a birth, but looking at the extremes, every birth can range somewhere from a C-section to an unassisted homebirth. Where a woman falls on the continuum will depend on her confidence, attitude, actual or perceived health, social conditioning, past experiences, opinions, values, and priorities, and where she falls on *The Birth*

Pyramid can indicate what type of birth she will seek. Each couple must decide what course of action to take and whether they are willing to take responsibility for their decisions and actions.

It is hard to make the case for a couple to have an unassisted homebirth if they have major fears about childbirth. Intuitive "gut" feelings may be telling you one thing, while your logic and reasoning may be steering you in another direction, while severe problems throughout the pregnancy may signal that you need a physician's care. This is not a failure on your part, but simply an indication that you may need the help of an experienced caregiver.

In the case of one spouse being ready for a homebirth and one opposed, remember that you have almost forty weeks to prepare. It may be smart to have a back-up plan for the delivery in case you are not able to go through with an unassisted birth. No childbirth experience should occur under extremely stressful circumstances, because increased stress levels could mean a longer, more painful labor and an unsafe birth.

Couples who are not confident about taking responsibility for an unassisted homebirth should probably not attempt it. Those who are overly concerned with what others think may not have the courage to do something as unconventional as unassisted homebirth. Lack of confidence or desire for approval from others can be worked on throughout the pregnancy, but the couple may have to conquer a lot of feelings of inadequacy to get to the point of feeling comfortable enough to attempt a DIY birth.

A final reason that someone should not have an unassisted homebirth is if it is being done for strictly selfish reasons. If the mother's health is poor and she would be better attended by medical professionals with access to equipment in a hospital, then she should not be giving birth at home without help. A birth event should not be an attention getting event or rebellious statement, or even worse, a situation which would put the mother's or baby's life in jeopardy.

5

"How Was Your Childbirth Experience?"

Thousands of women discover every day that they are pregnant. And then, the prenatal care they are given prepares them for a less than exhilarating childbirth experience. Unfortunately, they will go to a hospital to give birth and never know that the best circumstances for giving birth are found in nature, not science. It is assumed in our culture that when a woman gets pregnant she will select a doctor if she doesn't already have one and give birth in a hospital or birthing center.

When a woman is pregnant, the usual questions are: "Who is your doctor? What hospital are you going to? When are you due? Do you know the sex of the baby?" Instead, we should ask, "Are you going to have the baby at home or in the hospital? Why do you need an ultrasound? Are you doing your Kegel exercises? How are you preparing yourself mentally for the birth?" Our questions can help reshape the prevalent assumptions about pregnancy and birth, and can make others think about what they are doing and why. If a woman feels confident in her ability to give birth and if she feels that nature is on her side, why should she go to the hospital or why would she need a midwife attending her at home?

Many women recall their births as positive events, but more people are startled by the question, "How was your birth experience?" Such a question is often seen as irrelevant as long as a healthy baby and mother emerge from pregnancy and childbirth.

Our culture is much more concerned with the baby, the end product, rather than the process of being pregnant and giving birth. Pregnancy and childbirth are thought of, and often experienced as something to endure, to get through. It is much less common for a woman to describe her pregnancy as truly joyful and her birth experience as holy and serene. Parents refer to their baby as a miracle, but they dismiss the birth as unimportant.

The insincerity of "assembly-line obstetrics" contributes to a feeling of indifference during pregnancy and delivery. The mother-to-be learns to hold back emotions during routine appointments, where the medical personnel are just doing their job. The birth itself is often routine to the nurses and hospital staff, and women who do not have problems describe their births as "uneventful."

A birth event is permanently imprinted on couples brains. The birth experience will be remembered by the couple for a lifetime, yet often forgotten by everyone else within six months. What stays with us for the rest of our lives is all in a day's work to a medical team. Cindy Earley-Steinke reminds us that,

> You can't go back and do this birth over again. Ten years from now, this birth will only be a vague memory to the ex-neighbor or co-worker who pressured you not to do it [unassisted homebirth], but you'll still have your child and your memories...*forever*. You have the most to gain (and lose), so you two are the only ones whose opinions matter.

The choices we make

How we face birth is similar to how we face life. If we approach birth with confidence and flexibility, we probably approach jobs and relationships the same way, and if we are afraid of childbirth and rely on experts, we may lack the ability to set goals and make decisions. Women who avoid an uninhibited birth by seeking control through drugs or a C-section may shy away from the ambiguities of life. Childbirth experiences are the result of choices we make during pregnancy.

Reliance on technology

Pregnancy and birth are dominated by technology. As awe and excitement for technology increases, compassion and respect for the pregnant woman decreases, her opinions and comments being viewed as less reliable than electronic equipment. People are proud of their ability to master technology, and there is no incentive to strive for a natural birth. Many doctors assume that a woman has not kept an accurate account of her menstrual cycles, so in estimating the due date, two or three ultrasounds may be performed during her prenatal care. Blood tests to check for various sexually transmitted diseases and AIDS are routine.

While doctors and patients make decisions based on tests results, the danger is that most of these tests are not 100% accurate. Some couples feel pressured into making an abortion decision based on tests such as the alphafetoprotein (AFP), the chorionic villus sampling (CVS) or amniocentesis. These tests may not be conclusive and false positives are commonplace. Even though certain known and unknown risks are involved during ultrasound, and other procedures, many people believe that the tests and equipment used during their pregnancy and birth are completely accurate.

Patients who rely on technology are prone to laziness. People do not have to approach their health in a preventative manner. Most women do not know, accept or want to bother with the basics of their fertility. They prefer to depend on artificial contraceptives, which is more technology. Many OB/Gyns do not spend much time educating women, but act as suppliers. The education is often limited to a product's basic use and side effects—whatever can be explained in a ten minute office visit. Valarie Nordstrom, publisher of the "New Nativity II", a newsletter for do-it-yourself homebirthers remarked that

> women are encouraged to take birth control pills to suppress hormonal cycles throughout childbearing years. Then at menopause, they are encouraged to replace naturally diminished hormones. Manipulation of the female body extends nearly a lifetime!

Many Americans escape from life's minor pains and sufferings with pharmaceuticals, more technology. We rely on technology as a way of life. During labor, all eyes on the electronic fetal monitor rather than the mother's comfort level. It is no wonder women are somewhat unimpassioned about the childbirth process.

Drugs and why we should avoid them

Drugs carry risks and are harmful to the unborn and newly born. *The Five Standards for Safe Childbearing* and many other resources present facts about drugs that are used to ease the pains of birth. Women are willing to take chances with their unborn because they are not fully educated about risks, so they place their comfort above the health of their baby. Some drugs used in childbirth cause permanent damage in children. Psychiatrists have labeled disorders and attributed the causes to traumatic births, which almost always occur at the hands of doctors who use an assortment of drugs during a surgical or heavily intervened birth.

Drugs dull the sensation of birth, causing neither pain nor pleasure to be experienced in its entirety. The loud and intense noise that laboring women often make during natural childbirth is embarrassing or misinterpreted by medical practitioners, just as a three year-old child witnessing a sex act might perceive the event as painful. Adults perceive childbirth the same way because they do not understand or accept that birth is and can be pleasurable. In the absence of drugs, a mother nearing birth will often make noises comparable to orgasmic moans. The birth release is a combination of pain and pleasure. Adults misinterpret this ecstasy as agony and seek to block a true, full expression by the laboring woman. The more often drugs are used during birth, the less likely women report peak birth experiences.

Women focus on pain and discomfort rather than view pregnancy and birth as an opportunity to encounter their female sexuality at a deeper level. They take drugs to alleviate pain, and in the process, they destroy the possibility of feeling pleasure. If people realized that a birth experience could result in orgasm, they might consider striving for physical ecstasy rather than escaping pain.

Helen Wessel and others attribute postpartum depression to the absence of a birth climax. Women who are not fully awake and aware cannot feel the release after the baby is born.

> This climax is essential. A mother who has missed it and had a passive, frigid birth, due to anesthetics, local injections, or hypnosis, still is emotionally in a state of expectancy. She looks at her child, but experiences no euphoria, no sense of exhilaration. (Sousa 1976: 88)

Diana Korte and Roberta Scaer caution that when a woman takes drugs during birth, the body and brain are not able to effectively function and recover from the birth.

> Biologically, our bodies want to finish labor and give birth triumphantly, with our senses intact. Nature offers endorphins, too. Hard exercise, whether in labor, vigorous walking, or tear-provoking laughter, increases levels of these natural, narcotic-like painkillers in your blood. Endorphins are found in the placenta and are released in both mother and baby through labor, nursing, and skin-to-skin contact. One researcher has found that the mother's endorphin level after a cesarean birth is lower than after the exertion of an unmedicated, vaginal birth. (Korte 1990: 37)

Doctors assume women want to escape from pain and fear. There is basically no discussion by doctors about fear;

there doesn't need to be with the drugs and interventions that they prefer to use during labor and delivery. Unassisted homebirthers work through the issues of pain and fear and may encounter only minor pain.

Those who choose unassisted homebirth are not fearful of birth. Instead, they prefer to channel their energy towards reaching a healthy brain-body outcome rather than turning to drugs or surgery for birth. They know enough not to tamper with the brain. Friends and relatives opposed to unassisted homebirth often have a fear of childbirth which contributes to the view that the couple lacks common sense and the ability to exercise sound judgment. How is it that someone is irresponsible if they purposely avoid harmful drugs so that they can respect and enhance the brain's performance, without aid?

Physical pain and fear

Childbirth in the hospital is filled with everything that increases pain: tension, an uncomfortable birth position and a cold or foreign atmosphere. Fear contributes to pain and muscles become tense. The uterus strains as more pain is felt. Many women tense their whole body rather than concentrate only on the pelvic floor muscles. I saw a woman shortly after she gave birth who appeared as if she had been in a fight. It turned out that she had popped several blood vessels in her face. No one told her that pushing should be focused in the lower part of her body rather than face muscles.

> Experiments with animals that do experience pain in childbirth show that in certain species, drugs given to remove pain alter behavior toward the young after birth.... In all cases these animals rejected their newborns and refused to mother them.... Another theory of the use of pain is that it may serve in some way to keep mothers alert during labor and in the period immediately following delivery. In terms of muscle usage labor is fantastically exhausting, and it may be that pain counteracts the sensations of fatigue. (Macfarlane 1976: 34)

In humans, there are at least two contributing factors to the sensation of pain. First there is the nerve message to the brain following stimulation or damage to some area of the body. Second there is the state of the brain when it receives the message, and this is affected by cultural expectations about pain, previous experience of it, anxiety, fear, fatigue, and expectations about the outcome of the pain. If you hit your finger with a hammer, pain predicts a bruised finger. In labor, pain predicts the birth of a baby. (Macfarlane 1976: 35)

Permission and pressure

Listen to people describe their birth events and you will hear words describing a certain passivity or bondage.

> They wouldn't allow me to move around even though I was uncomfortable; They had to leave the electronic fetal monitor hooked up; They had to induce me; I'm glad I was in the hospital; I needed to be there. My baby was almost 10 lbs.; The doctor had to use a vacuum extractor and I ended up with a fourth degree tear; I had to return the baby to the nursery because of visiting hours; The nurses seemed to be so busy getting the measurements of the baby that I didn't want to interfere with their job.

During labor, it can be intimidating to ask for what you want or need. There is pressure to conform to the policies of the hospital and practices of the obstetrician. Nurses and doctors who deal with a majority of women who desire drugs during labor assume that all women want to escape from pain, and people are sometimes pressured into receiving drugs that they do not need. Many do not know what the possible effects are. Indeed, some women do not view C-sections as

---

If you are distressed by anything external, the pain is not due to the thing itself, but to your estimate of it; and this you have the power to revoke at any moment. —Marcus Aurelius

major surgery, but just another way of having a baby. In fact, some have been delighted that they were able to resume sex sooner after a C-section than a vaginal birth.

The threat of malpractice is constantly on a doctor's mind and the obstetrician would rather protect himself than be concerned with the couple's needs, making for a subservient relationship between patient and doctor causing the patient to feel that she must respect the doctor and therefore go along with his plan.

"Birth plans" are becoming more popular. The couple states their desires and intentions for labor and delivery and provides a copy to the doctor and hospital before the due date. Another copy is usually given to the hospital staff during labor. The copy will usually get filed and not taken seriously because the power relationship is in the medical hierarchy's favor. Birth plans are more likely to be followed if the patient is assertive and persistent or has a doula at her birth. The expectant woman must talk about her intentions so that medical personnel will know she is serious about what she wants.

Greed and control by birth attendants lessen a couple's experience of the birth. If power is given away freely, someone will be there to accept the power, make decisions and exert control. Instead of having a staff to serve you, you may feel as if you have to ask permission to do what you want. You may feel uncomfortable asserting yourself to take back some of the control you need for a satisfying birth.

Denial

Women know intuitively that there is something missing from their birth experiences, leading to a silent sadness after birth. Discussing experiences with other women becomes a reporting process. Complaints are exchanged and the couple may focus on the significant high points, but nothing seems to matter as long as the baby is healthy. Then the chatter quickly moves on to the postpartum adjustment and development of the newborn. "Are you getting any sleep?

How much does the baby weigh? Is he a good baby (meaning, does he sleep through the night?)" Many women do not even remember the details of their births and what drugs they were given.

The process of giving birth does not seem to be important enough to make changes. When the issue is brought up, there is a lot of denial associated with it because most women do not enjoy their childbirth experiences. Man-imposed interventions will continue as long as the idea that there is a better way to have babies remains unknown.

Subservient patients are the supporting actors in their birth events, while the doctor plays the starring role. Instead of trying to break away from the cultural way of giving birth, a vast majority of women go to hospitals and put up with the doctor's way of delivering babies. Most deny that a problem exists because (1) How would they fix it? And (2) If patients knew how to fix it, would they really want to? Change takes effort and requires a commitment to new ways of doing things.

Postpartum depression

I have talked to and read about hundreds of women whose birth experiences revealed a lingering emptiness because the birth occurred outside a couple's intimate space.

Birthing in the home among loved ones does not include separation, drugs, and unfamiliarity—three key factors that contribute to initial postpartum depression. At home, the mother's emotional stress is often lower and the baby is usually content. New mothers are tired; they may feel ambivalent—rather then depressed—about their new family. Aidan Macfarlane, author of *The Psychology of Childbirth*, describes a study where some level of depression occurred in 60 percent of hospital deliveries and in 16 percent of home deliveries. Depression following unassisted homebirth is probably lower than 16 percent, but more research is yet to be done in this area.

Give me a few adjectives to describe three months postpartum following your homebirth. If the birth story you wrote about was not your first child, how does this postpartum period compare with earlier birth experiences?

Kirstina Wimberley feels so strongly that the postpartum attention in this country is very lacking and offers many ideas and insights.

> This is definitely a part of childrearing that needs to be addressed in politics. Health insurance companies should offer a paid doula service for child abuse prevention and physical and mental health for new mothers. Most people don't have friends or family to help after a birth. We had friends bring one meal and family bring another. My family lives in Europe so I definitely needed more help with cooking, cleaning and shopping. Our two older kids, age ten and eight when our third child was born, are actively involved in survival techniques and could be self-sufficient if they had to. Since my two older children were from a previous marriage, my third child was my current husband's first child. He got a greater understanding of the work and healing involved after birth and actively took part. Fortunately, he has a job with a progressive organization that paid him three weeks paternity leave after each birth. I don't know how people handle it without that support.
>
> I understand domestic violence is greater than ever because the financial burden, poverty, and stress in families because of children is outrageous. The best part of my three homebirths was that it cost nothing. Where would we be if we had to pay for our children's entry into the world on top of everything else? Homeless, maybe. *[or childless. That's exactly what couples often choose—the least expensive and least burdensome route as they strive for self-fulfillment/ indulgence]*.

> Tired, happy, sad. It was hard dealing with my two year-old (who was mistakenly shut outside during the final moments of birth, left to hear the shouts and moans of birth). I felt as if I had wronged him terribly.

In some ways, euphoric and awesome. In other ways, stressful.

It was harder because Cody was the third child and a lot of work needed to be done. We used cloth diapers and no dryer. There was a lot of food preparation and cleaning.

My postpartum experiences have always been fine; a bit busier with each additional child, but pleasant.

Joyous, romantic. What a great thing we had to brag about. I was on "cloud nine" for months. I would smile every time I thought of my husband, scared out of his wits, catching his baby and putting him in my arms. How I loved to brag!

Postpartum is very difficult for me. I had horrible after pains (even after using Afterease tincture) for three days. With so many children, I was obliged to be up taking care of meals, laundry and other household duties much sooner than I felt ready. This set me back. I became quite depressed and cried a lot. I did not receive the nurturing I felt I needed to gradually recover. After four months postpartum, I was still not fully myself.

Continuity. There was no disruption in our lives. The new baby flowed into our family. No trip home from the hospital, no paperwork, no hassles, fears or worries. As magnificent an event as it was, it fit like a puzzle piece. I think this was especially important for our two year-old daughter.

It was a smooth transition: loving, caring, supportive, nurturing. I found my breastfeeding relationship to be a much easier experience and transition than I did the first time around.

Satisfied would be one word. We didn't need to depend on some M.D. who didn't even know us, to deliver our baby. We could do it ourselves. Other words would be exhilarated and blessed.

Energetic, excited, devoted, affectionate, and of course, tired. This postpartum was not as bad as people warned me it would be, considering we had twins. I had mentally prepared myself for the twins, long before they were born, and so they have always been a joy to our family.

Every time I look at our "DIY baby," I am reminded almost daily of her wonderful birth. When I look at my other children, their births have sort of left my mind. My postpartum period has been one continuous blissful experience—an inner smiley face attached to my heart, even though I may feel tired from a baby who wakes up every three hours or overwhelmed from the stresses of life.

From talking with others who have had DIYs, I think that DIYs have a powerful effect that carries them through other difficulties in life. A DIY is a major accomplishment." If I can do this, I can do anything." Increased self-esteem provides a resiliency and helps to cope with other difficulties or sufferings that may come their way.

Midwife delivery versus unassisted birth

I have heard so many beautiful homebirth stories, both assisted and unassisted, yet when it comes to satisfaction, there is definitely a difference between midwife-assisted and unassisted births. Couples often begin their birth experiences in hospitals and evolve to unassisted homebirth. Because the level of satisfaction is so much greater among those who give birth without attendants, it is rare for such couples to revert to hiring a midwife for their next birth, or using any other form of attended birthing.

Conflicts are bound to happen in human interactions, but a husband and wife who are so intimately involved know their own comfort level, and are better equipped to deal with differences that arise. When you introduce a third party, the dynamics become a little more complex; communication breakdowns often occur; and expectations differ.

I have spoken with many people who had midwives at their birth and were very satisfied, yet they felt they could have done it unassisted. Sometimes, midwives show up late or want to be in control of events, but unassisted homebirth reduces the chance for human relationship problems and medical interventions. When you ask a couple who has had an unassisted homebirth how their childbirth experience was, you are bound to hear a testimony that reveals a contentment not often heard in traditional birth stories, because unassisted homebirth involves no schedule, permission, or pressure from outsiders.

It's up to you

Doctors, midwives and hospitals have goals for birth. Have you set any goals for your birth? There are millions of women who will never experience the beauty of unassisted homebirth for the simple reason that they continue to relinquish their power to make their own choices.

Instead of mothers giving birth freely and naturally, obstetricians deliver babies medically, robbing women of their natural role in birth. The unnecessary drugs they take will dull the pain and the senses, and minute traces of drugs will be passed on to the baby possibly jeopardizing the very first moments of parent-child bonding. As the new family begins to build a lifelong relationship as a family, they will feel relieved that their hospital birth experience went so well, never knowing that one of the greatest opportunities to have a peak experience has just escaped them.

I've been promoting this 22 years—and *not one* couple, that I know of, has ever said, "I'd rather have people surrounding me next time instead of just my husband."
—Marilyn Moran, 1996

If children are not born well, the whole of society suffers.
— David Stewart

6

Birth Conformity

The Major Deterrent To Unassisted Homebirth

Conformity is safe and easy. When we do something different, we risk being labeled as outcasts or loners. Because our need for belonging is strong, unassisted birth does not appeal to many people.

While those who believe the myths of childbirth are more likely to conform, even those who do not accept the myths of childbirth conform to traditional birth practices if their need for security is stronger than their desire to live according to heartfelt beliefs and intuition.

The myths of childbirth

Birth is a simple process, but because of our fears, we do not accept the fact that birth is uncomplicated and safe. Perhaps there were problems that warranted specific attention, but what originally started out as genuine concerns have been embellished. Myths are sometimes perpetuated by those who know the truth. So misconceptions must be challenged by educated and courageous people in order that the process of change can begin.

Myths come from misinformation and ignorance. Actions are based on beliefs and often become habits. When cultures adopt commonly held beliefs and habits, they then influence birth practices. The nine myths of childbirth are an example of "cultural conformity," the major stumbling block to change. People who refuse to accept new ideas that challenge the myths will have difficulty accepting unassisted birth.

Myth #1: Pregnancy and birth are abnormal.

Physicians and their patients have all too often considered pregnancy and birth an abnormality or illness. The goal of pregnancy is to treat any discomfort and rid the body of the abnormal, ill condition. Heartburn and nausea often accompany pregnancy, but these discomforts are temporary and expected as the body undergoes major changes.

When the fetus is seen as a foreign intruder, it is hard to rejoice about pregnancy, making childbirth thought of as painful and unnatural, as if the body were not designed to give birth. Those who believe this myth then become overly cautious and try not to cause further disruption. While the mother is taught that she must accommodate this burden state, she then begins to view what should be a time filled with joy and anticipation as a personal sacrifice, a mere condition threatening a selfish lifestyle. Some women avoid physical activity, sexual pleasure and make other changes because they think pregnancy and birth are abnormal.

Abnormal cases require professionals to solve problems and develop treatments. They seem to test the limits of science, by looking for problems. Since everyone has minor discomforts, it is easy to label every pregnancy as some type of problem; prenatal appointments become focused on abnormalities through various tests and screenings. The abnormalities of pregnancy and birth include not only rare defects, but man-imposed interference such as fertility drugs and vacuum extraction deliveries.

> Mother, coached by father, behaves herself, while doctor delivers the baby. —Barbara Katz Rothman

*Myth #2: Technology always benefits pregnancy and child-
birth.*

A woman who does not view herself or the baby as the
center of her birth is inviting technology to be a major part
of the event. Technology is available in the hospital in case
there are problems. For the majority of women who do not
have problematic births, it seems that technology is employed
for fun (and profit). The misuse of technology sometimes
results in unnecessary inductions and C-sections, often resulting in premature babies.

People imagine birth without technology. They assume
childbirth methods were primitive and dangerous. The danger was caused not by the absence of technology, but by inferior personal hygiene and other factors. Perhaps there were
more deaths without technology, but far too many infant
deaths today are caused by advanced science.

Dr. Edward H. Hon invented the electronic fetal monitor (EFM) and intended it to be used only during difficult
labors. Now, the EFM is used routinely, requiring that
women be in a restricted and often uncomfortable position
during labor. The EFM is used to make important decisions,
which often lead to unnecessary interventions. "Oh, no, the
baby is in distress; we must do an emergency C-section."
Here is what Hon stated about his own invention several years
later after its widespread implementation: "Not all patients
should be electronically monitored. Most women in labor
may be much better off at home than in the hospital with the
electronic fetal monitor." (Armstrong 1990: 131)

There are at least three opinions on the safety of ultrasound. Many say it is perfectly safe, while others say that we
don't know the effects of ultrasound, and some cite evidence
that ultrasound is dangerous. The American College of
Obstetrics and Gynecology, the American College of Radi-
ology, and the US Preventive Services Task Force all recommend *against* routine ultrasound screening of low-risk pregnancies.

Technology is beneficial when it is used to aid difficult situations where it is impossible to rely on human means. Unfortunately, technology is often used to direct the birth event. "Fun tools" have replaced "outdated" or "archaic" means of monitoring a pregnant or laboring woman. We continue to move away from human contact and natural birth as we increase the use of technology.

Myth #3: Birth is usually unsafe: death is a possibility.

Anything can go wrong with the mother and the baby. Death may occur during childbirth. People obsess about a remote possibility, but their fears do not reflect reality. Generations have managed to reproduce without a massive infant or mother mortality rate.

The belief that birth is unsafe has contributed to current obstetrical practices. To ensure that birth will be safer, doctors feel the need to manage birth in a controlled, predictable manner. The baseline for a successful birth is that the mother and baby emerge from the ordeal alive. Many people believe birth must be attended by a physician in a hospital to prevent against the possibility of death. While people are concentrating on all the things that can go wrong, they cannot see all that is going well.

A doctor, trying to dissuade a woman from an unassisted homebirth said, "Your baby could die." The woman countered, "Babies die in hospitals all the time." "That's different," the doctor replied. And the woman said, "Not really. They are just as dead."

Perhaps the same group of people who worry about death in childbirth do not fret about the possibility that their plane will crash, that they will contract a disease from store-bought food or that they will get into a fatal car accident. While death is a highly unlikely result of childbirth, it is more common in hospitals than at home. Newborns exhibit breathing difficulties more frequently after medicated hospital births than they do in unmedicated births at home. Hospital nurseries are filled with many more unhealthy babies, percentage wise, than babies born at home.

> Compared to home-born babies, hospital-born babies are six times more likely to suffer distress during labor, eight times more likely to need resuscitation, four times more likely to become infected, 30 times more likely to suffer permanent injury, and their mothers are three times more likely to hemorrhage. The high risk is in the hospital. (Balizet 1996: 141)

Those who believe that birth is unsafe question the common sense of those who have given birth without assistance. Common thoughts include: "How can you be so irresponsible?...You were lucky that everything turned out all right....I'd rather be in the hospital so I can be assured that they will take good care of me." Planning an unassisted homebirth implies that a couple will consider safety. Very few people purposely seek unsafe outcomes. A person who is unthinking is irresponsible. Going to the hospital ignorant is much more unsafe and irresponsible than being fully prepared for a birth at home.

Whether they are born in a hospital or at home, the majority of babies are born alive and healthy.

Myth #4: Birth is an emergency.

If birth is an emergency, why do many doctors show up for delivery at the last possible minute? The labor and delivery staff in a hospital calmly go about their business while the mother is waiting around to deliver her baby. It is not until the baby is about to be born that the birthing room dramatics begin. The doctor may order commands when to push. His instruments are wheeled over to him and the anesthesiologist suddenly appears. The entire delivery room staff seems to act as if a major crisis is about to occur, making the mother feel as if it is an emergency.

> The crisis nature of birth was retained from the medical model, and childbirth, as practiced by the Lamaze, prepared-childbirth instructors, continued to be defined in terms of medicine rather than motherhood. It is the homebirth movement that presented the genuine challenges to the medical model. (Rothman 1992: 94)

The out-of-hospital births which get media attention are those that are not planned. A recent headline in a local paper told the story of a couple who was speeding to the hospital and had the baby in a car. Everyone was relieved that things turned out favorably. People expect a major problem in the absence of a professional and attribute success to luck. Our biology works in certain ways for certain reasons; there is no luck about it.

Myth #5: Professionals are needed to deliver babies.

If birth is abnormal, unsafe and an emergency, then a professional must manage the situation. "Birth moved into hospitals in large part because doctors believed it was a surgical event." (Rothman 1994: 284) Patients allow doctors to make most decisions for them and submit to C-sections and unnecessary interventions.

The growing popularity of the "man-midwife" or barber surgeon and his instruments in the 1760's were probably not needed to "improve" childbirth. The professional emerged not because of his superior skills, but because of the power of men to convince women of (1) the dangers of childbirth and (2) the incompetence of female midwives. Couples were eager to pay men for their services since they had higher social status and demanded high fees. Professionals slowly replaced the female-midwife. A lot of knowledge began to be lost as these new birth salesmen moved into unfamiliar territory. They could easily conceal their birth injuries and mistakes with scientific jargon.

Obstetricians and midwives often approach childbirth as a business. It is not unusual for birth to become a mechanical-surgical event, complete with medication and physical restraint. Birth decisions are based on the convenience of the doctor rather than the parents. When you sign up with a doctor or midwife, you are signing onto their regulations and restrictions; their choice of hospital comes before yours.

Many people believe that the doctor or midwife has the best interests of the patient in mind. This may or may not be true, depending on the particular attendant. Patients believe that because they pay experts, the experts' judgment is flawless. Many women do not see themselves, but their doctor or midwife as the center of birth. Professionals are not *needed* to bring about a birth. Most babies emerge when they are ready.

Myth #6: Birth is unbearably painful.

Rather than prepare for birth naturally and lovingly, women fear a big baby passing through the vagina. The assumption that childbirth is extremely painful is accepted as a fact, and since it is perceived as true, the experience of pain often accompanies the birth. The father is asked to be distant from the whole experience and to focus on trivial breathing exercises with his wife. Many couples attend weekly lessons on how to breathe, only to forget them when they get to the delivery room.

Related to this myth is the idea that you need drugs to make it through the delivery. Drugs are readily available and can alleviate any amount of pain a woman may have. Sedatives and narcotic drugs are used to squelch complaints.

Physical pain intensifies not only because of the actual pain experienced, but also based on a woman's perception, ability to cope with pain, and level of emotional support. Hospitals do not provide much emotional support. People she has never met before will be present at her birth, making sure she is hooked up to the EFM. On a busy shift, the nurse will have to go from room to room to check the EFM results, leaving the woman alone to stare at the clock.

Birth is defined by pain: what to do about it rather than how to avoid it or how to work in synchronization with it.

Without drugs, the first stage of labor may be more painful, but the second stage, the pushing phase, will be less painful and more manageable by the woman. All a mother really needs is reassurance and human compassion.

Fear and pain go together when it comes to childbirth. Grantly Dick-Read said that fear influences the muscles which cause tension and anxiety. Pain intensifies and doctors are there to relieve that pain.

> Civilization and culture have brought influences to bear upon the minds of women which have introduced justifiable fears and anxieties concerning labor. The more cultured the races of the earth have become, so much the more dogmatic have they been in pronouncing childbirth to be a painful and dangerous ordeal....If fear can be eliminated, pain will cease. (Dick-Read 1959:6)

"Of all our physical functions, only lovemaking is as much influenced by thoughts and emotions as labor. The way the mother thinks and feels affects the way she gives birth." (Jones 1987:5)

Myth #7: Childbirth is scary.

Through the birth experience we come to terms with who we are and how we deal with stress and uncertainty, because birth is an opportunity to test our physical and emotional limits. While many people live their lives with a sense of busyness and flight from self, some people are so terrified of spending time alone that they occupy their time with activity. Those who fear birth flee from themselves, but it is in the quiet moments that spiritual and psychological truths are discovered.

Fear comes from an inability to trust the body and nature, and women's magazine sales thrive on an inferiority complex which leads women to think they need to aspire to some ideal body. The pressure to improve weight and muscle tone is not motivated so much by health reasons as much as it is by psychological reasons. Indeed, some people do not even enjoy their pregnancies and at the eighth or ninth month, they are looking forward to having the baby so that they can shed those "unsightly pounds and get back to normal."

A poor body image contributes to inhibitions, often accompanied by shyness, modesty and embarrassment. When a woman expresses fear to her doctor, she is questioning her confidence and ability. Most doctors will not ask a woman why she doubts herself, nor will they tell her that birth is normal and that there is no reason to fear it. Instead, doctors often accept the woman's self-assessment as fact. They do not help build a positive body image for pregnancy and birth, but rather let the fear spread into pain and treat the pain in the delivery room.

Insecurity contributes to the myth that childbirth is scary, so drugs are used to minimize fear and inhibitions as well as to reduce perceived or actual pain. Because of this, not only do women miss out on satisfying birth experiences, but low self-confidence regarding the ability to give birth often carries over into the beginning days and months of parenting, leading those who are petrified of childbirth, also to be frightened of parenting.

If we think and act as if birth is scary, we will ignore our inner intelligence, which tells us that birth is not to be feared. We will rely upon experts, never realizing that we are experts.

Myth #8: The C-section was necessary.

"Thank God for the C-section. I needed it." Maybe so and maybe not. Although some women are grateful for the special medical attention that brought about the birth of their child, others are disappointed with themselves or their doctors.

Many people accept the idea that every birth is a potential C-section. A baby in "distress," in breech position, or too big to come out vaginally often prompt C-sections. Many women are grateful for the C-section of their 9 lb. baby because they are fearful when they imagine a vaginal birth of a big baby. Many others are relieved to have a C-section when the EFM reveals that the baby's heart rate stopped or that labor was not progressing.

Research indicates that the true need for C-sections applies to five percent of the pregnant population, but (depending on the doctor and hospital) approximately 25% of women end up with C-sections. A friend of mine told me of a hospital with a 50% C-section rate.

> The medical establishment states to the public, as well as to the students in their medical schools, that the increased cesarean rates are for the benefit of mothers, babies and families. The data do not support this claim. (Stewart 1997: 56)

Many C-sections are preventable. Proper prenatal habits and attitude during birth combined with an unhurried attendant may be all a woman needs to avoid a C-section.

Myth #9: Women need episiotomies, especially with the first-born.

Some episiotomies are needed and others are performed because of the preference or routine of the doctor. The "need" for an episiotomy is, after all, determined by the doctor. Many women tear even after they have had an episiotomy and many others have long and difficult recoveries from episiotomies—probably worse recoveries than if they had torn.

Many women are not taught perineal massage and do not have warm water with oil applied to the perineum to prevent tearing. Lying in a supported supine position in the birthing room does not help matters. In fact, many childbirth educators have presented data which show that a squatting position at delivery reduces tearing by an additional ten percent. If women knew how to prepare their bodies (during the prenatal period) and followed a few simple procedures during birth, there would not be a need for an episiotomy.

I have heard of only two or three women (out of hundreds) who have experienced significant tearing during a planned unassisted homebirth, regardless of the size of the baby.

How you can have a satisfying birth in spite of the myths:

1. Change what you think about birth and you will change your experience of it.
2. Ignore pessimists and complainers. Surround yourself with people who have had fulfilling births.

When birthing in the hospital:

3. Do not allow anyone to define what childbirth should entail. You can choose how you want your birth to go by setting goals, planning, and asserting your desires in the delivery room.
4. Arrive at the hospital well into labor. You may feel more comfort (and less pain) at home. There will be less time for overuse of technology.
5. Realize that the birthing room drama is often exaggerated and that most births are not true emergencies.

Social conformity

Myths adopted as truth by the majority lead to social conformity, which has at least two levels of expression: compliance and identification. Compliance occurs when people are motivated by the desire to gain reward or avoid punishment. Scowls, frowns, laughter, criticism, ridicule, complaints, refusal to communicate and threats are forms of punishments.

The last thing a laboring woman wants to do on a hospital bed is to be non-compliant with the staff. Being physically and emotionally vulnerable, the mother seeks approval from the hospital staff. She wants a smooth delivery—one that appeases the staff. Unfortunately, the medical personnel do not really care about physical and emotional vulnerability; they are there to do a job. And their job is to comply with policies and procedures.

We are influenced by individuals and groups we admire. Strong identification with others leads to imitating their behaviors and, in some cases, adopting their desires. This can result in a "loss of the self," leading to an increase in the need to conform. When we do not fulfill others expectations, we risk disapproval and increased isolation.

Security is assured when we conform with the expectations of others. Any personal doubts about identity are silenced. There is a high price involved here: a thwarting of one's own life by giving up spontaneity and individuality. We may be alive biologically, but we are emotionally and mentally incomplete.

Because of social conformity, many pregnant women have birth experiences which are not of their own volition, but are defined by others. Popular magazines and books carry little information on homebirth. Reluctance to have an unassisted homebirth is not so much a problem of actual risk as it is a mindset that precludes couples from considering unassisted homebirth. Many assume that they are not the "type" to have a homebirth, while others wonder if it is legal or how they would go about it. People who visualize the birth of a baby as costing over $5,000 and view birth as a process which requires specialists, find it hard to imagine that amateurs could take the place of trained experts.

"Ultra-conformity"

Knowing yourself, accepting yourself and feeling comfortable with yourself all contribute to psychological and physical health. Some people fear—and avoid—an inner familiarization. Growth of the self is impaired if you're concerned with status, following, or being like others.

Some degree of conformity is necessary in a modern, civilized society, but conformity in its extreme, or "ultra-conformity" hinders cultural change. Ultra-conformists who know that certain changes can make a positive impact in their lives still prefer comfort over improvement. We might see an improvement in prenatal habits and marital relationships if the masses practiced unassisted homebirth, but as long as people are unwilling to make "nonconforming" decisions, there will not be a surge in unassisted births.

Ultra-conformists fear controversies, visibility or being different. They do not act or make conclusions based on their own perception, nor do they allow themselves to experience what they truly feel. They often avoid disputes and become anxious in situations which require self-awareness and self-discovery.

Abraham Maslow says that the only way ultra-conformists can achieve safety and order, free from threat or anxiety, is through orderliness, predictability, control and mastery. If conformists can proceed into the future on the basis of "well-tried" rules, habits, and modes of adjustment which have worked in the past (and which they insist on using in the future), they feel safe. But they experience deep anxiety when they face new situations, when they cannot predetermine behavior, when they do not know the acceptable form. Gradually, conforming people lose touch with their real feelings.

Individuals experience little fulfillment when they disregard their wishes and capacities. They strive to achieve safety and status and to overcome their desires and gain victory over their natural surroundings. Even though they are separated from nature and others, they appear to be in harmony with them.

These conforming persons do not use their own resources or experiences, but take direction from experts, authority figures, and traditional guides. Somewhere along the way they have given up their actual identity and become submerged in acceptable group behaviors. Having been rejected by others as unique, independent people, they may never discover their talents or find their place in the world.

Spontaneity does not come easily to ultra-conformists, causing predictability, planning and safety to contribute to a serious demeanor, and the innocence and spontaneity of childhood to be seen as undesirable in adulthood. As they

---

The danger of the past was that men became slaves. The danger of the future is that men become robots. —Erich Fromm

progress from childhood to adulthood, they form facades for self-protection, by adopting behaviors and attitudes that will fit in with society.

Life should be about unpeeling your mask and finding out who you are, what you like and dislike, value and believe, and then living that way. Old age is often a return to the innocence and spontaneity of childhood with the added benefits of wisdom and life experience. An unassisted homebirth gives you the freedom to be uninhibited, with your mask totally off—a frightening situation for ultra-conformists.

Confrontation and encounter

Conformists are motivated by the need to avoid emotional pain and discomfort rather than by seeking fulfillment. In fact, *confrontation* and *encounter* actually help establish authentic relationships, but conformists avoid them. A confrontation is a meeting between two people in conflict or controversy. They are often face to face and they may or may not remain together until their feelings of divisiveness and alienation are resolved. A pregnant woman may have to make several confrontations with her medical providers to accomplish something different from what they are used to doing.

Presenting a birth plan to the hospital requires assertiveness and is confrontational for the mother, just as informing others of your plans for an unassisted homebirth may turn into a defensive session with people who hold opposing viewpoints.

An encounter is a sudden, spontaneous, intuitive meeting with another person in which there is a sense of harmony and communion. Because birth is sexual and loving, a birth encounter between a husband and wife alone is a love encounter. An intimate unassisted homebirth renews the relationship, while a birth in the presence of strangers does not set the stage for such an encounter.

An encounter can be a creative experience, causing a dropping off of conventions so that one enters into the reality of a situation in terms of the conditions and requirements intrinsic to that situation. Openness and relatedness are part of the encounter, characterized by a free and open play of attention, thought, feeling and perception. Even though the openness and intensity of interest in any one encounter may range from the grave, the serious, the absorbing, and the tantalizing, even to the playful and fleeting, every encounter is an opportunity for couples to learn something new about each other.

Risks of being a conformist

While conformity is a fundamental, natural tendency of human beings, social norms do not always serve us well, often causing us to react in ways that encourage imitation and discourage deviation.

> Most people are not even aware of their need to conform. They live under the illusion that they follow their own ideas and inclinations, that they are individualists, that they have arrived at their opinions as the result of their own thinking—and that it just happens that their ideas are the same as those of the majority. The consensus of all serves as a proof of 'their' ideas. Since there is still a need to feel some individuality, such need is satisfied with regard to minor differences; the initials on the handbag or sweater, name plate of the bank teller, the belonging to the Democratic as against the Republican party, etc. (Fromm 1956: 11)

A growing trend in the obstetrics business is the merging of practices, leaving women with no guarantee which doctor will deliver her baby and, in some cases, what hospital she will go to. It depends who is on call during her labor. In many parts of the country, she will select her doctor and be encouraged to meet all the doctors in the practice. After all, it does not matter to the practice which doctor delivers the baby. Women hold onto false hopes that their preferred doctor will deliver their babies, and discuss—with positive acceptance—the fact that a different doctor actually attended their birth. They never even realize that they are treated as "consumers." Ultra-conformity stops them from questioning the system or demanding changes.

Risks of being a nonconformist

Expressing unconventional opinions leaves you vulnerable, by putting your identity at stake as a result of openly declaring yourself through your commitments. Commitment requires courage, and you must be willing to face being considered unsuccessful or just plain wrong. In committing yourself you forfeit your opportunity to blend in with the mob, to tag onto the coattails of a winner, or to switch loyalties without anyone else noticing. Being committed opens you up to being challenged, accused and ridiculed.

Nonconformity can be lonely. Almost everyone has a need for belonging and companionship, making it frustrating when you look around and notice that very few people share your opinions and values. It takes considerable strength to stand up for unpopular beliefs and to combat the loneliness or anxiety that accompanies nonconformity.

Characteristics of nonconformists

Here are a few characteristics of people who lead healthy, nonconformist lives: they speak their minds; they do a lot of experimenting; they say no to others occasionally in order to say yes to themselves; they are forever learning. Regardless of their age, such people live on the edge of new knowledge, new fields, and new discoveries. They spend time with people who encourage their nonconformity.

It is a rare gift to find people who are loyal and give you space to be yourself. But you learn to value them highly and to give them the same space they give you. They are always creating something and often stay off the beaten path. They like to be with children and think less about people's opinions while being more spontaneous. They often have dynamic, interesting personalities, resisting conformity and developing some small eccentricities as part of their journey to independence and self-confidence.

The mass of men live lives of quiet desperation. —Henry David Thoreau

7

Preparing For An Unassisted Homebirth

Safety

The American Medical Association, midwives and child-birth educators cannot deny that birth at home is safer than in the hospital. From the Mehl Study, which proved a higher safety rate for birth at home, to The Farm statistics, homebirth is safer. As new technology is used during birth and as new drugs are introduced to alleviate pain, interventions will increase and create a greater gap between safety at home versus safety in the hospital.

The fixation on unassisted homebirth as unsafe stems from the belief that the hospital is a safer place to deliver and that birth needs to be managed by skilled attendants. The problem is that most people falsely believe that the technology used in hospitals will be the exact amount necessary for the individual patient, no more or no less. It also assumes that the attendant will apply the skills needed for a healthy, natural birth. In reality, more problems occur in the hospital where a skilled attendant does not have a loving relationship with the birthing woman, than occur in an unassisted homebirth where the birth occurs in the context of a reasonably prepared loving couple.

Some situations in the hospital are labeled as problems, which precipitate treatments and decisions. Medication complications and prematurity are not safety issues at home.

> The perinatal mortality rate for planned home births is very low indeed—3 or 4 per 1,000 compared with 9 to 10 per 1,000 births as a whole. Moreover, two of these three or four deaths are unavoidable wherever the baby is born, because the baby is extremely preterm or suffers a congenital handicap that is incompatible with life. All that birth in a high-tech hospital might do is delay death by a few days or weeks. (Kitzinger 1991: 51)

What you can do

There are certain precautions a couple needs to consider before embarking upon an unassisted homebirth. Prepare for possible problems. If you intend to have an experienced friend come to your birth, prepare for her absence. You will need to consider equipment and supplies. Supplies will depend on personal preference and your preconception about how safe birth is.

Write down or mentally review your plan for action in case of minor or major problems. There are risks involved and measures that need to be taken for a baby who is not breathing or a mother who is hemorrhaging. Couples need to know what to do in the event of shoulder dystocia or placenta previa. What would you do if the baby was stillborn? If you think you will feel more comfortable using medical equipment, be certain that you know how to use it. An oxygen tank takes special training to operate and a stethoscope or fetoscope is useless if you cannot determine whose heart beat or what sounds you are hearing.

Since 1940 at least a million babies have died in American hospitals who would have lived were it not for the doctor dominated maternity system that dictates the Standards for American Childbirth. —David Stewart

---

If the father performs a vaginal exam to check cervical dilation, he will need to be able to make a precise calculation. If the couple decides to rupture the membranes, they should know what they are doing and why, rather than assume it is necessary or desirable because doctors often do it. It will not be necessary to take all of the sterilization precautions that are followed in the hospital. The baby will be fortunate to enter the world into kind, loving hands in a natural, clean setting rather than slither into the hands of a masked and gloved stranger dressed in a scrub uniform.

My safety concerns

For the most part, I trusted my body to carry and deliver a baby without major problems. After all, it had not failed me on four other occasions. My confidence increased as my knowledge about handling problems increased. I was never fearful of cephalopelvic disproportion (CPD), a long labor with slow dilatation of the cervix, or a long second (pushing) stage, because none of these situations surfaced in my other births. I was concerned about a breech baby, prolapsed cord, cord wrapped around the neck, placenta previa and shoulder dystocia, but my worries were eliminated once I discovered what to do in those situations. In the final weeks of pregnancy, my major concerns were perineal tears and postpartum hemorrhaging.

I had never heard of perineum massage before my fifth pregnancy. In the eighth month, my husband tried it a few times, but it was uncomfortable, so we stopped. Our plan for the birth was to fill a crock pot with water, add olive oil and keep it on a low setting with washcloths nearby. Bob would apply the washcloths when necessary to see that my perineum was flattening out and pink. White skin tissue would indicate poor blood flow and likelihood of tearing. I also decided that I was not going to push until the baby's head was out. I believed that the baby would enter the world when it was ready. My research, opinion and past experience was that the baby made its descent on its own time, not mine. I would simply facilitate its emergence.

I was concerned that I might hemorrhage and that I would not have pitocin or some other drug to stop the bleeding. I thought about making arrangements to have some medication at home, but I realized that I would not feel comfortable determining how much medication to give myself and then to actually administer it if I needed it. I had previous births with heavy bleeding afterwards. The reason for the bleeding was important to know, not just the fact that I hemorrhaged after the placenta was delivered. Since the heavy bleeding resulted because the placenta was pushed, pulled and extracted from me within ten minutes after birth, we decided that impatience and disrespect for the placenta would not be tolerated in our homebirth.

Since I knew we would be letting nature take its course, I did not fear that I would bleed to death in some freak accident of childbirth. I let the placenta remain in me for forty-five minutes after birth and noticed that only one-half cup of blood followed. Medical employees with obstetrics experience warned me that a woman's uterus is unreliable with five or more births and that hemorrhaging was to be expected. Because their birth experiences were based on hospital procedures with women in various health conditions, their safety concerns were not relevant to my situation.

Although I read about Shepherd's Purse and other remedies for stopping bleeding, I considered the most extreme life-saving precautions. Would I be willing to do any of them if I needed to save my life in a split-second? If the answer was yes, then I felt courageous enough to have an unassisted homebirth. If I was not willing to do something extreme, then I had no business attempting an unassisted homebirth. The most extreme measure I was willing to do was eat part of my placenta if I hemorrhaged. One midwife with twenty-five years experience has treated hemorrhaging in many ways. In 100% of her cases, severe bleeding stopped within four minutes of ingesting part of the placenta.

We live within fifteen minutes of a hospital and knew that we would not be alone in an emergency. I felt safe about our birth at home because I had a higher level of trust and preparation going into the birth event than ever before. The same technology and intervention that can help save a baby's life in the hospital, can also be responsible for a greater probability of something going wrong before it is born.

Is prenatal care necessary or desirable?

Each woman has the right to take care of her pregnancy how she wants, just as she has the right to care for herself when she is not pregnant, whether it be her diet, personal hygiene or exercise habits. When women are urged to get prenatal care, it usually means visits with a doctor. Women who seek prenatal care from a lay midwife, skilled friend or conduct it themselves are accused of being irresponsible. Ironically, the self-reliant group of women who seek alternatives follow better nutrition, exercise and other prenatal habits because they have taken the responsibility to ensure a more comfortable and safe delivery. On the other hand, women who get prenatal care from obstetricians may have never heard of Kegel exercises or perineal massage since they have abdicated responsibility to a group of professionals who do not view these preparations as important.

Optimum health is a goal of any woman who is pregnant, regardless of where she will give birth. Women who choose to have an assisted or unassisted homebirth are much more likely than the general population to take good care of themselves throughout their pregnancies. Prenatal care among women whose stories appear at the end of this book were varied. Whether they sought out assistance from a doctor, midwife, husband or friend, all of the women took full responsibility for their pregnancies.

Kirstina Wimberley admits that her preoccupation with finances and arguments she was having with her husband caused additional stress during her pregnancy. They were in the process of building a house. The only formal prenatal care she was interested in was a visit or two with a midwife. Her family is athletic and they enjoy basketball, riding bikes and taking walks on their 60 acres of property. She credits her healthy pregnancy to a solid vegetarian diet, but admits to indulging in chocolate.

A chiropractor soothed the discomforts of pregnancy for Shannon McNear of Goose Creek, South Carolina. She never saw a health care provider and exercised three times a week.

> At the beginning of my pregnancy, I did step aerobics and weight machines, but cut back to walking 1-1/2 miles each session. My nutrition was better than most women, but could have been better. I've experienced blood sugar problems with past pregnancies, but I felt pretty good throughout my pregnancy once I passed the morning sickness stage.

Kim and Frank Pratt's first child was delivered by an obstetrician in the hospital. Because the doctor had diagnosed her with an "incompetent cervix," he stitched the cervix at five months when she went into pre-term labor. Their second pregnancy brought them back to the doctor even though they were planning a midwife-attended homebirth. They did not inform the doctor of their plans, and the midwife had no objection to the Pratt's using a doctor for back-up plans. "I was fearful that my OB would be mad that I did not go to the hospital. I now know that is ridiculous and I have to remind myself that I'm a consumer and adult and can do what I want."

Kim was dissatisfied with the OB/Gyn not only because he had a reputation for inducing women whose babies ended up not being fully developed, but also because he believed in performing internal exams at many of the visits toward the end of the pregnancy. Although he recommended bed rest, she felt good and was active. Kim followed excellent nutrition habits to provide her with a high energy, upbeat attitude.

Sheila Stubbs, mother of six, believes in minimal prenatal care from a physician and that women should focus on good nutrition. She felt comfortable showing up three or four times to be weighed and measured to appease her doctor. Herbal teas and refusing to take drugs for some of her problems resulted in a healthy pregnancy and baby.

Patricia Kohl, mother of seven in her early forties, believes that prenatal care with a doctor or midwife is unnecessary. She checked her blood pressure weekly since she experienced a lot of swelling and tried to maintain proper nutrition. She ate plenty of fish, made whole wheat bread, but admits that more fruits and vegetables should have been ingested. She did not get much exercise, and felt it did not effect the delivery. Swelling, heartburn, carpal tunnel syndrome and frequent nosebleeds were other discomforts she experienced.

> I took excellent quality supplements during my last two pregnancies: multivitamins, extra vitamin C, red raspberry, nettles, alfalfa, dandelion, herbal calcium and herbal iron (yellow dock). Also, six weeks before my due date, I took evening primrose oil and blue and black cohosh tinctures to facilitate labor.

Cindy Earley-Steinke, of Lynchburg, Virginia, was very thorough during her prenatal period. With the help of her husband, she weighed herself regularly, took her blood pressure, fundal measurements, palpitation and urinalysis. She saw her family doctor three times for urinalysis, hematocrit, or just a general check-up. An ultrasound was requested when she suspected twins.

> I did pelvic rocking, squatting, walking, tailor sitting, relaxation practice and 'legs apart exercise' daily. I followed the Brewer diet and felt great. Although I gained 59 lbs., I lost 35 one month postpartum. I contracted a rare pregnancy-related rash called PUPPP (pruritic urticarial papules and plaques of pregnancy), which I also contracted at the end of my first pregnancy.

When Judie was pregnant with her twins, she was very excited. She read many books about the importance of taking care of a pregnancy with multiple births. Nutrition, exercise and rest were very important.

A multiple pregnancy requires plenty of fluids. Six months into the pregnancy I went into labor. I didn't even know it until the midwife attached a fetal monitor to me. I had to go into the hospital for IV feeding. It was frightening, but it ended well. Once again, I disliked my midwives and some of the comments that were made. I had enough, and decided to take matters into my own hands. A homebirth was the answer.

Charity Gregson of Washington performs prenatal care during each pregnancy.

We do our own prenatal care. This includes blood pressure checks, pulse, fetal heart tones, fundal height, and vaginal exams toward the end of pregnancy. After our decision to do our first DIY, we purchased a *William's Obstetrics* textbook, a blood pressure cuff, and a stethoscope so we could monitor the pregnancy and be more aware if any complications should arise. I felt great during all pregnancies. I enjoy being pregnant and have never had a day of morning sickness.

Wendy Bunkelman talks about preparing for her midwife-attended birth:

With my second child I saw our local lay midwives and received excellent holistic prenatal care. Nutrition was my number one priority. I ate high protein, many whole foods and incorporated some herbs into my diet. I biked close to five miles a day with my eldest on back. As a whole, I felt great.

Your spiritual base

Because an unassisted homebirth is such an awesome responsibility, many couples rely on a spiritual foundation. The moment of childbirth is a rare moment in life where we realize that we are not in control of life. It can be very emotionally stressful and physically painful. Those who have a strong need for control may prefer to have drugs or a C-section. Those who are able to embrace uncertainties and sufferings often seek spiritual support.

Spirituality includes beliefs, attitudes, meditations, prayer or practice of a particular religion. Whatever the case, a belief in God or a higher power can provide a tremendous source of strength.

Insecurity often accompanies the moments of conception, birth and death. It seems that God is operating at a very personal level during those times. By turning the heart, mind and soul towards Him, you can invite His love to fill you with the power to accomplish anything. A well-grounded spiritual foundation allows people to welcome birth and death. Spirituality can put you at ease and peace rather than in a state of fear, shock or flight.

Those who have worked hard to develop a strong spiritual base during peaceful times in life will have help during difficult moments in life. Those who do not gain strength from spiritual avenues come to the unassisted birth process with one less resource.

Author and born-again Christian Carol Balizet makes an excellent point when she says,

> In the medical system, what is available is human knowledge, human reason, human effort. It's what the Psalmist calls, 'horses and chariots,' the arm of flesh and the interventions of man. Very few Christians will admit to having more faith in the medical system than they have in God, but very few are willing to trust Him without the medical system. I think the time is coming when we will have to recognize it's an either/or situation. (Balizet 1996: 62)

Your mental outlook

We choose how our birth will go regardless of where it is, when it takes place, or who is present. Attitudes, intentions, and state of mind all have a major effect on the birth as well as other events in our lives. Someone who is extremely fearful of childbirth will probably end up having a birth where she takes minimal responsibility and makes little effort.

While many people think you need to be mentally prepared for an unassisted homebirth even before you get pregnant or during the early part of pregnancy, that is in fact not true, nor is it necessary to live life trying to have full mastery over an event that has not taken place. Growth occurs when you respond to events as they unfold, and as trust and courage improve, fear and doubt will disappear. This takes time and effort and is an evolving process.

Those who go against the norm must have courage to stand up for what they believe. As you progress through life's journey, you develop more strength. Forty weeks should be adequate time to prepare for an unassisted birth. One couple may not have the courage to have a homebirth until the thirty-ninth week of pregnancy. Another couple may be fully confident about a DIY even before they conceived a child. If each couple was psychologically prepared the day before the birth, they would both be mentally ready. The only difference is that one couple spent more time in mental anguish than the other.

> There seems to be a relation between anxiety, overt or covert, and the length of labor. Uterine dysfunction may also be associated with concealed anxiety. Harry Bakow found that mothers who were anxious during pregnancy and who expressed more concern over the course of their pregnancy more often had babies who got into distress at delivery. Recent studies suggest that women likely to have complications during childbirth are those who during pregnancy manifested a negative attitude to the pregnancy, showed concern for the condition of the child, saw their employment as being disrupted, listed a greater number of contacts with women who had complicated pregnancies, and described their own mother's health as poor. (Macfarlane 1976: 18)

> We are what and where we are because we have first imagined it. —Donald Curtis

Whether a woman decides to give birth in or out of the hospital, her labor will often last as long as she expects it to. Many women prepare themselves for a thirty-hour labor at home and end up with a thirty-hour labor.

In *Visualizations for an Easier Childbirth,* Carl Jones poses five questions we should ask before choosing a place to give birth: "(1) Am I the center of my childbearing experience in this place? (2) Am I fully in charge? (3) Is this the place where I want to begin a new family? (4) Is this really the best place to make the transition to life outside the womb? (5) Do I receive the emotional support I deserve in this place?" (Jones 1988: 42) Finding honest answers to these questions can give a woman the positive mental outlook she needs in order to have a rewarding birth event.

Questionnaire responses

How was your frame of mind regarding fear, anxiety and tension during the pregnancy? How did you cope with it or prepare yourself to deal with fear, if you experienced it?

Wendy Bunkelman: Exercising and relaxation exercises helped to release any fear, anxiety or tension during my pregnancy. I absorbed myself into books to become as informed as I could and tried to maintain good communications with my partner.

Jeanie Haas: During my first two unassisted homebirths, I studied scripture with my husband and was so relaxed. I had no fear. I just knew that God would be faithful. Because our son (third unassisted homebirth) lived for only one month, I had some apprehension about postpartum issues.

Cindy Earley-Steinke: I had a lot of anxiety about how my husband would handle things. I nagged him all the time to read more books! It really bothered me for a long time until I realized that the baby was coming whether he was prepared or not. Of course, when the time came, he was very prepared and wonderful!

Keith Steinke: I had some anxiety also. I read the books that Cindy and I thought would be best. Although I didn't read as much as I should have, when the time came I had a calm inner peace. I worried how we would handle it. But again, when the time came, I was calm.

Shannon McNear: I felt occasional "attacks." I believe that fear is the biggest single cause of problems in labor. Besides the relaxation exercises for simple tension, I guess I could say that my "secret" is dealing with it in the spiritual realm: prayer, scripture, praise. Fear is the opposite spiritual force of faith and must be dealt with as such.

Troy McNear: Anxiety that things would go smoothly. Dealt with by prayer.

Sheila Stubbs: Pain: Birth seems "easy" the day after the birth, but during the last weeks of pregnancy, I remember there was pain and knew that I must face it. Health: What if something goes wrong? What if they rush me to the hospital, accuse me of being irresponsible, take my baby away, put my children in a foster home? Baby: What if my "luck" runs out and my baby is unhealthy and they blame me and accuse me of being an unfit mother and...

Bert Stubbs: I just let it happen. Well, yes there were fears, but I just let it happen.

Patty Kohl: During the early part of the pregnancy, I had a great fear of another miscarriage which exhausted me. I felt things were more normal once I felt the baby move. Then towards the end, I did fear the pain of labor, which I dealt with by lots of reading.

Rick Kohl: I was concerned about her swelling—that something would go wrong and ruin our plans for a DIY birth. As the birth approached, I became a little nervous and was hoping that everything would go fine. As soon as my wife went into labor, I wasn't scared or nervous at all.

Kirstina Wimberley: No fear. Total self-confidence and trust in the process, self of God (Buddhist).

Jesse Wimberley: No fear during pregnancy. I had a sense of anxiety about what to expect at birth. I spent most of the pregnancy studying books on delivery and actual birth stories. I followed pregnancy development with Kirstina.

Charity Gregson: As we made plans for our first DIY, I was worried a little about the legal aspects of having our baby at home with no medical assistance. I had not heard of anybody in recent history doing it. Although I suspected that there wouldn't be a problem, I was very hesitant to mention our plan to people for fear that some medical person would get wind of it and really chastise us. I've since discovered that there are no laws regarding how a woman gives birth. [*author's note: Each couple may want to check their state laws regarding birth, birth certificate requirements and other concerns.*] My main anxiety during the pregnancy was of the possibility of complications. I prepared myself by studying the different complications and their warning signs. I highlighted the most common complications and their remedies in our *William's Obstetrics* textbook for my husband to review. We also had our vehicle ready for an emergency trip to the hospital located five miles from home.

Judie: When we finally made the decision to homebirth, we told no one but our two children who knew to keep it quiet. Fear and questions were constantly rearing their ugly heads, but I knew that from the beginning I would be challenged with doubts. I did a lot of praying and reading of

God's Word—morning, noon and night. The great thing about this is that once labor began, I was at complete peace.

Peter: Initially, I really did not have much anxiety, but once I learned that we were having twins I began to feel a little worried. As I read about others peoples' experiences and focused more on the promises of God in the scriptures, my concerns subsided a great deal. I truly felt a new sense of peace from Christ. Whenever I began to think or project about the things that could go wrong, I would get worried again. I found that talking over the promises of God with Judie and meditating on some key Bible verses would put my concerns at rest.

Who should I tell about my plans?

Being a nonconformist in a conformist world requires energy. You can isolate yourself from conformists, but this is not usually desirable or possible. You can mentally choose to detach yourself from others or you may decide to persuade some people of your plans. If you are seeking approval from everyone, you may find yourself lying or not revealing your true intentions. For the many different people in your life, you will come up with what is suitable for you.

The most important people who should be communicating are the mother and father. You may need to let the other children in your family know, depending on their ages, how much participation you expect of them, or if they will witness the event. You will have to decide how much of your plan you wish to reveal to other adults living in your home. It would not be fair to expect certain people to witness or help at a birth without having had time to prepare.

Couples may want to tell their parents of the upcoming homebirth. Some families often discourage independent thinking, and members who stray too far from what is expected, are often punished with disapproval, ridicule, judgment or hostility. Because such independent thinking is sometimes seen as a violation of the family structure, responsibility and loyalty, those who rebel because of their personal standards often do so at the expense of familial criticism and ostracism. So if you think family or friends will applaud your discovery that an unassisted homebirth is a far superior way of giving birth, remember that internal happiness is not as easily rewarded as fitting in. There are those who would like to impose certain conditions of worth and prefer relating to you only if you are in an approval-seeking mode.

Every time you decide to do something apart from the norm, others intentionally or unintentionally put you on the defensive, causing you to explain all the benefits associated with your choice. While you are wasting your breath in a persuasive argument, their hearts are not really open to your point of view; they are either nosy or fascinated. Some people are genuinely interested and impressed, while others dismiss you as unreasonable and fanatic.

Your support network

Regardless of who you tell about your birth plans, you will probably want some type of support network. This network could simply be you and your mate. If you plan on having the child without the assistance of the father, he should at least be in support of your plans since it is his child too. Some people prefer to surround themselves with many people who are in favor of their plans so that they can talk freely and frequently with their friends. Others are content to be alone and know that many of their friends and relatives are present in spirit. Because the period from pregnancy through birth is an emotional time for a woman, a cushion of comfort surrounding her is vital to her well-being.

Modern medical care devalues emotional and spiritual support, regarding technology as the most important support that women need. Some medically minded workers are opposed to labor support people and view them as a threat. Profits from the birth business come from liberal use of drugs, surgeries and technology. Those who favor drugged births do not appreciate a labor support person "intervening" in their domain by talking a woman out of an epidural.

Professional labor assistants such as doulas (Greek word meaning "in service of") and monitrices (French word for "a woman who watches over attentively") have comforted many women in hospitals and birthing centers. They provide continuous care and support during labor and delivery, often reducing the labor time and need for medical interventions. They may not be needed at an unassisted homebirth where the mother is already very comfortable in her own setting with her lover. However, some women would not consider laboring without a doula or monitrice.

When planning an unassisted homebirth, you may have to decide who will be at your birth to act in a supportive or motivating role, or to clean up afterwards or watch the other children. You may prefer someone to take the other children out of the home during the birth. If another adult is at your birth, be sure it is someone with whom you have a comfortable friendship and similar philosophies. A close relative or lifelong friend has no business being at the birth if they are petrified or against what you are doing.

Back-up plans

Many people who have unassisted homebirths fully trust the process, while others feel security in having a doctor ready to meet them at a hospital on a moment's notice. It depends how fearful the couple is and what they perceive as requirements for a safe delivery and healthy newborn. Past pregnancies and experiences may play a major role in the level of back-up plans. A friend of mine paid to have an ambulance park in her driveway during the birth of her daughter.

Leaders have the courage to begin while others wait for that inopportune moment.

Did you have any emergency, back-up plans?

Hospital is ten minutes from here.

No.

Nothing, except to call the local rescue squad if an emergency did occur.

Not really, just prayer. That seems foolhardy to most, but that was our position.

Yes, we had my OB/Gyn's number on hand and a route planned to the nearest hospital.

Several people had been asked if they'd be available if necessary. That way we knew at least someone would be able to help.

Yes, we notified the rescue squad of our plans and had them put up a notice on their bulletin board. We did not arrange anything with a doctor; they are very unsupportive here. We had Shepherd's Purse in case of hemorrhage and clamps in case of an unusually tight cord.

We have the hospital phone number posted near the phone. We discuss with those present with us during early labor what each person's job will be should an emergency arise. Depending on the severity of the complication, someone will call the hospital so they can prepare for our arrival. While the call is being placed, the others present will be helping to transport me to the vehicle, which was already prepared for a rush to the hospital. If the complication is life-threatening, someone will call 911 for an ambulance.

Yes. We would travel 140 minutes to the CNM who attended my first birth. Otherwise, an ambulance to the local hospital.

Birth and delivery tips

1. What are some techniques, strategies or practices you

can share that helped you have a smooth delivery?

Visualizations of flowers opening up, giving birth to new seeds.

We really didn't have any special technique. Our desire was to rest in God, and trust Him to bring forth our baby.

Do not have anyone present who has a negative attitude or is not completely comfortable in the situation. Any anxiety in the room may be felt by the others present and could cause the mother to become tense.

Faith and trust in God. I know that without Him I couldn't have had such a wonderful homebirth. Peace and joy was all around us as the babies emerged. We verbalized God's promises to each other as a reminder of His faithfulness to us. I stood and gave birth as Peter took hold of his new twin sons. It was a wonderful and awesome experience.

Each woman has to find the technique that best helps her to deal with her labor and delivery. I instinctually chose the hands and knees position which helped to relieve the pain I was feeling in my back and helped me concentrate on each contraction with slow, deep breathing. In between contractions I found the bathtub filled with hot water helped to completely relax me and prepare me for the oncoming contraction.

Confidence.

Be confident in what you are doing. Be well prepared both physically and psychologically. Do a lot of reading beforehand and pray for assistance, as we are all weak. God is our strength. Stay close to each other and husband and wife should talk a lot about the coming birth.

Spiritual preparation first as a way to deal with fear and other anxieties. Trust that birth was designed by God and that it works.

I took PN-6 and blue cohosh toward the end of pregnancy and when my water broke during labor.

Stay on your feet when in labor. Walk faster, breathe slower with each contraction. Rather than thinking, "Oh no, here comes a contraction," think, "Oh yes! A good strong one. Ouch, yes, that's what I want!" Kissing relaxes mouth and therefore cervix. During transition, wrap your arms around hubby's neck and hang from him—it allows your hips to widen. Allow yourself a certain number of transition contractions and countdown to remind you how short this difficult stage is. Soaking in a tub relaxes muscles and helps loosen skin around perineum. Walking and squatting during labor and birth speed things up. Use a crock pot for hot compresses.

2. What birth supplies did you have ready?

Clamps, scissors, betadine, towels, vinegar, padded sheets, bulb syringe, cayenne pepper, herbs.

Lots of disposable pads, towels, cord tie, scissors, flannel pillowcases (great for wrapping and drying baby), syringe, scale, Depends pads for mom postpartum. A plastic shower curtain makes a great mattress protector.

The whole birth kit.

We ordered a kit: plastic bed sheets, gauze pads, almond oil for perineal massage, sterile gloves, underpads, thermometer, sanitary pads, elf cap, povidone-iodine solution, squirt bottle, bulb syringe, alcohol cord clamps, hydrogen peroxide, sanitized sheets and towels, baby clothes, bowl for placenta, laborade.

We purchased the items suggested by Marilyn Moran in her book *Birth and the Dialogue of Love*. This consisted of sterilized scissors and baby shoe strings, plenty of towels, newspaper, baby caps, nose cleaner and diapers. Along with these, we added drinks and foods rich in iron, as I am anemic. Soft gospel music, tape recorder, camera and large plastic to cover our bed.

We order our supplies from an Oregon-based company. For our births we use sterile surgical gloves, bulb-suction syringe, underpads, antibacterial handwash, plastic cord clamps, Gentian violet and alcohol prep-pads for cord care, and the book *Emergency Childbirth, by* Gregory White. We also use the stethoscope to monitor fetal heart rate and the blood pressure cuff to monitor my BP. I used maternity sanitary pads with the comfortable cotton-mesh panties, also ordered with our other supplies. Our last birth happened so fast that we did not have our supplies accessible. We used the bulb-suction and the cord clamps.

Underpads, bulb syringe, old towels and washcloths, 2 plastic-backed sheets, white shoelaces and scissors, water for baptism if necessary, olive oil, 2 sterile gloves, basin for placenta, baby clothes, Shepherd's Purse tincture, Smooth Transitions tincture.

Pads, towels, cord clamps and scissors. Bulb syringe, clothing for baby, prepared a lot of extras like the olive oil for perineal massage, gauze pads. We prepared a lot of stuff, but in retrospect, our needs were very simple.

A couple of old, cheap, plastic tablecloths to protect the floor. White shoelaces and a pair of scissors. Several old, soft towels and receiving blankets that can be thrown out if stained. A large green garbage bag. Ultra-super, heavy-duty maxi-pads.

Crock pot, washcloths, perineal massage oil, hot water bottle, sheets, towel, shower curtain, Chux pads, scissors, cord clamps, herbal cord care, Shepherd's Purse, baby clothes and diapers, baby scales, tape measure, thermometer, blood pressure supplies, fetoscope, gauze pads, basins, *Emergency Childbirth,* phone numbers, written notes, penlight and a clock.

3. Did you do any internal exams to check dilation or effacement?

7 couples said no.

Yes, but my husband wasn't really certain about what he was feeling.

Yes, self-checks.

Yes, but we were unable to determine what was going on.

Yes. My husband learned to estimate the amount of dilatation and effacement with our first DIY. He does a vaginal exam 1-2 times per week the last couple of weeks of pregnancy and as needed during labor.

4. Did you experience any fear, anxiety or tension during the birth?

Mother: No
Father: I experienced intense fear—panic—when Cody unexpectedly began to crown without any early signs of labor progression, such as no mucous plug lost, no water broken. This was followed by a complete sense of relaxation and profound calmness as his head presented.

Mother: Near the end of my fourth DIY on 4/1/96, I began to feel anxious because pushing didn't seem to be doing anything. In retrospect, I realize that the baby was "high" (according to my midwife one week prior to the birth). I forgot all about that during my long pushing stage. The baby was born in her bag of water, so my water never broke.

Mother: No, I felt calm and assured that everything was moving along perfectly.
Father: Yes, since I was seeing everything as it was happening I felt anxiety when my first son's leg got stuck for a few seconds. Then it came down on its own and I was really relieved! At first I wanted to rush it along by moving it, but I'm glad I didn't intervene.

Mother: I experienced some anxiety during transition and my second stage only because I was alone. I knew the baby was coming soon and was trying to figure out what position would be the best for me to deliver.

Mother: During my first DIY birth I had a fleeting thought of "Will I be able to do this at home?" During the other births I had no worries because we kept careful records of the baby's well being and I knew that I had done it once already.

Mother: No, none at all. I had full confidence in Frank's abilities.
Father: I felt that during the birth, I was "in the groove." Everything was flowing, the energy surrounded the three of us with white light.

Mother: I was somewhat afraid of the pain as labor progressed, but mostly I was very relaxed and happy—grateful the time was finally here.

Mother: Yes, fear of the pain. I dreaded each contraction.
Father: No.

Mother: No. I'm quite relaxed and trusting, a little excited the time has come; anxious for it to be over soon, though.
Father: I'm always worried when I see them come out purple. You don't know whether they're dead or alive.

Mother: Yes, right after transition. My urge to push was not overwhelming for some time and it was difficult and confusing figuring out how to work with my body.
Father: The only fear I had was when I tried to check dilation and could not figure it out. The rest of the time I felt I was calm and was there for Cindy.

5. How did the physical pain (or pleasure) of your DIY compare to other births?

The pain of labor was about the same for each of my six births. My hospital births were also drug free and "natural," so I felt every contraction. The ability to move around during labor at home was the best pain reducer, as I had been confined to the lithotomy position in both of my hospital births. The euphoria I felt after my DIYs was so great that all labor pains were forgotten shortly after the births.

Once labor began I was not fearful and this is why I believe it went so well. The birth was too quick to remember, but I do recall the sudden widening pressure and feeling myself bearing down. The pain wasn't a discomforting "ouch," but more of a complex task that needed full attention and energy. I felt the Lord's strength taking over as I knew I could not have done anything without His help. I let God take over for I didn't know what was happening to this body of mine. He orchestrated the whole event and it went so well.

I think having been through childbirth before helped me to look at the pain as temporary. I always felt comfortable in my own environment and not threatened.

I felt the same outrageous, intense pain at transition. I felt very powerful that I could handle it. I did a ten minute birthing song to handle the sensation which opened up my vaginal canal.

They were all different, but being in labor in peace made things much more pleasant.

There was a lot more pleasure just because of the fact that I was at home. I was really happy to be having a baby at home. My labor was so short that I had little pain.

I felt more in control during these births and the pain of the contractions was intense, but seemed much more productive and definitely less erratic.

This was our fourth baby, and first homebirth. I felt less pain than the first two, but more pain than the third baby. The third baby was a slow induction—just enough to nudge labor along. The pressure was incredible, and although this was my biggest baby, delivery was less painful than the others.

Very little pain; very little pleasure; *very* romantic.

There was more pain with pushing because I wasn't working with my body as well. First stage labor was much less painful.

6. Was your length of labor shorter than the other births? Estimate the length of labor for each child.

1$^{st:}$ not sure 2nd: 3 hours 3rd: 2 hours (DIY) 4th: 4 hours (DIY)

1st: 7 hours 2nd: 60 minutes 3rd (twins): 25 minutes watching water dripping from my amniotic sac with an additional 35 minutes of labor.

1st: 3 hours 2nd: 1 hour, 45 minutes

First 4 births were about 24 hours and the waterbirth was 12 hours from the first contractions.

1st: C-section 2nd: 12 hours 3rd: 30 hours 4th: 3 hours (DIY) 5th: 3 hours (DIY) 6th: 5 hours (DIY) 7th: 30 hours, but not intense (DIY)

My length of labor was very short with my second child (1st DIY). The first was four hours and the second was maybe twenty minutes. I think I slept through second stage labor.

Hard, intense labor was much shorter during our DIY births. In all seven of my labors, start to finish was always 7-9 hours. In our midwife attended births, I think the pain was worse because I felt I had to "be on my best behavior" and act as I should with a guest. This increased my fear and tension and the painful part of labor was longer.

Early labor was longer, while active labor was shorter. 1st: 30 hours labor (21 hours active labor) 2nd: 3-1/2 hours total, induced. 3rd: 9 hours total—slow induction. 4th: 1-1/2 days early labor and 4-1/2 hours active labor (DIY).

1st child: 21 hours, then a C-section. 2nd child: 28 hours VBAC 3rd: 12 hours (1st homebirth) 4th: 6 hours 5th: 3 hours (DIY) 6th: 3 hours (DIY)

1st child: 4 hours. 2nd: 3 weeks prelabor, 5 hours actual labor (1st DIY) The second was longer, but I felt it would have been shorter if I worked with my body sooner.

7. What would you like to do differently regarding the pregnancy or birth?

Next time, I'd like to skip the OB all together and I'd like to have more people at the birth. I'd like to have someone experienced in childbirth present so that it would take some pressure off Frank.

Not much. Maybe just have myself and husband there and no one else. At our DIY, a close friend was there for support and assistance.

More friends or a doula service to help after the birth so we can focus on the spiritual aspect.

Watch my diet more carefully and gain no more than 35 lbs.

My husband says there won't be a next time, but he said that after our 2nd, 3rd, 4th, 5th child. I'd rather have a DIY again, and I wish my husband wasn't so scared.

As far as the pregnancy or actual birth—nothing differently except to lay on the bed after the birth rather than the couch, since there is more room on the bed. Rick gets nervous after the birth and goes outside shortly afterwards to take out garbage and bury the placenta. I'd like him to stay with me longer.

Next pregnancy, I will drink 2% milk instead of whole milk. And at the next birth I will be less afraid to push when all signs point to it.

Nothing. I feel as though I have reached the epiphany of my childbirth experiences. I would like my next labor and birth to be a little longer, but that is nothing I can control.

If blessed with another pregnancy, I would like to record the birth on a tape recorder. The first cries and gasps of air from my newborn would be wonderful to sit and listen to over and over. As the years roll along, memories like these are great to hold onto.

During all four of our DIYs my husband guided the head out with his hands. My babies come out very fast, and since they are generally large babies, my husband is afraid that I will tear when the head emerges. He is very adamant about me not pushing but to let my body push the baby out. However, he has never had the sensation of every urge in your body telling you to push. The last few minutes of labor are very intense for me as my husband is very insistently telling me not to push, while I am trying to comply. The next time, I just want to push without a word from him. If I tear, then, oh well. I tend to think that I won't since I had a 10-1/2 lb. boy without tearing.

---

10 reasons not to take risks: (1) we've never done it before (2) nobody has ever done it before (3) it's too radical a change (4) the staff will never try it (5) customers won't like it (6) we're not ready for it (7) you're right, but (8) good thought, but impractical (9) we'll never be able to do it (10) it's impossible. —Sheila Murray-Bethel

PART II

Joy and Triumph

8

An Unbreakable Bond

Michael and Sarah sitting in a tree
Michael and Sarah sitting in a tree
Michael and Sarah sitting in a tree
K - I - S - S - I - N - G
First comes love, next comes marriage
First comes love, next comes marriage
First comes love, next comes marriage
Then comes baby in a baby carriage.

Remember that song from elementary school? The songs children sing often represent an ideal for which to strive, and show that children do not view marriage and babies as a burden. Songs and stories are part of the socialization of a people. Western societies depend on strong nuclear families, but they do not just happen; they take a lot of hard work. Mature love, strong marriages and satisfying birth experiences contribute to confidence in adulthood and a love for children, leading to competent parenting and a rich, rewarding family life.

Tolerance of alternative lifestyles is important in a culture with diversity. However, as tolerance increases, so does complacency about the importance of the traditional family unit. Many people do not devote themselves to keeping their marriages and families intact as if their life depended on it. Instead, couples are apt to dissolve their unions when they grow apart or no longer love each other. Divorce is common-place and children must learn to adjust to single-parent households and step-families.

Unassisted homebirthers represent various family struc-tures portrayed in society. Some babies are born to unmar-ried mothers and others are delivered by an older child or former boyfriend. Some married couples who have shared an unassisted homebirth have divorced years later. Whatever the situation, birth should always be about love and unity, not divisiveness.

The ideal family situation is a loving marriage where joint decisions are made regarding conception, birth and parenting philosophies. Optimal attachments are made and bonds are formed when there is a sharing and full involvement between husband and wife. The goal is to build a strong family be-ginning with the birth of a child, allowing a happy, fulfilling marriage to evolve and grow. The mystery of femininity is taken away with artificial contraceptives and bottlefeeding just as the mystery of childbirth is taken away with medica-tion and surgery. Husband and wife homebirth is a way to celebrate the mystery of life and love.

It is not automatically true that marriage intensifies be-cause of an unassisted homebirth. Because the woman's ex-pectations and acceptance of her husband's behavior during the birth are critical, the husband's lack of involvement dur-ing the pregnancy can cause resentment among some women anticipating unassisted homebirths. Many women expect the fathers to be more enthusiastic and to read more about child-birth. In her preparation for the birth, the woman may have done extensive research, but the husband also must be pre-pared for anything and everything during the birth.

Men often share in the excitement of the new baby, but do not usually express their feelings the way their partners would like. The disappointments may carry over from the pregnancy to the birth and beyond if issues are not resolved. In this chapter, I will show how an unassisted homebirth can lead to a deeper love.

First comes love

Love involves a sharing of hopes and desires. Each partner wants his mate to be happy, healthy and successful. The other's needs are given higher priority. Two people seem to merge and enhance each other's sense of aliveness.

> True love involves making the other person a giver too. And both share in the joy of the new bond, the new level of being, the new sense of aliveness that is born between them.... True love is not blind. It is rather a special kind of knowing that reveals to us all at once, intuitively, the whole being of the other in a mysteriously lucid manner. (Imbiorski and Thomas 1969: 37)

Love involves risking. When you put yourself to the test of trusting and depending on your lover, your loyalty and respect increase immensely. There are few events you will experience other than unassisted homebirth that will lead you to trust each other more. Your child is living proof of that love and trust.

Next comes marriage

Love is perhaps most satisfying in a monogamous, lifelong committed relationship. It is in marriage where you will have the freedom to give and take. You will share joy and sorrow, as well as grow and change and share in each other's personality. In marriage, partners must take the risk of giving all that they are and all that they have—of pouring themselves out completely, without reservations. True lovers are no longer two persons; they have achieved a unique identity, together.

Most couples who decide to marry enter the marriage with the idea that it is a lifelong commitment of many promises.

Gifts of the Holy Spirit: wisdom, awe, understanding, reverence, knowledge, fortitude.

It is hard to imagine that one's love can be deeper than on the wedding day. For young lovers in the beginning stages of marriage or a relationship, there may be a lot of self-love and idealization. Each person may be projecting himself onto the other. There is a hint of selfishness that goes undetected. Love is in its infancy and at a more prominent physical than spiritual level. There will remain a void if a couple never progresses beyond this less mature, narcissistic love. A superficial or exclusively sexual exchange of sensations will bring about pleasure, but not true joy.

After a period of time, which varies among couples, imperfections emerge. The novelty passes and the "we" reveals a separateness, which requires each partner to examine how individual identity fits into the collective identity. A more mature union occurs when the soul and psyche lead the body. Then the personality is loved and new mysteries about the other person are discovered. The birth of a couple's first baby will be the first time that the lovers can observe each other in a brand new role, that of mother and father.

Behind every successful marriage and homebirth is a third force at work. To many it is God and to others, it may be called something else. Those who are open to receiving and expanding God's influence are allowing strong powers to work in their lives. Love is a means to a higher power and that higher power is a means to a greater love.

Many people have felt an inexplicable force that pulled them together before marriage. Those who believe that an outside force is at work during a couple's mystical attraction often feel that their lover is a gift, while others see their spouse as a possession that exists to fill their needs for happiness, physical pleasure or companionship.

Marriage is mainly about unity and indissolubility, which is achieved through fidelity and mutual assistance. A perfect union requires spouses to mature, accept each other and reveal to each other new depths and facets of themselves. Faith, hope and trust are needed for love to reach a higher dimension. Conjugal love is enriched by trials, sufferings and sacrifices. Marriage is about the deepening of love.

People set themselves up for disappointment if they expect something extraordinary from their mates. It is not your mate's purpose to bring you happiness. Not even the perfect love relationship with a lifetime mate will bring complete satisfaction if people do not realize that they are seeking something outside themselves, a sense of spirituality, God. True joy occurs when there is a link between the flesh, the mind and the Divine, in the presence of lovers and God. This is possible during an unassisted birth.

JOHARI WINDOW

	known to self	not known to self
known to others	I. OPEN	II. BLIND
not known to others	III. HIDDEN	IV. UNKNOWN

The "Johari Window," developed by J. Luft in 1961, is a concept often used in human relations training and management development. It is used to assess self-awareness by identifying known and unknown information to the self and others.

This model can be applied to marital relationships. An important way couples can deepen their love and attain a stronger union is to make new discoveries about themselves and each other. Interactions are easier when people know something about each other. Quadrant I, the open or public quadrant, represents behaviors known to the self and to others. Behaviors known to others, but not known to the self are referred to as "blind." Quadrant III represents those areas which are hidden; behaviors are known to the self, but not known to others. As you can see, Quadrant IV represents behaviors of which the self and others are unaware.

Although the four quadrants appear equal in size, the areas expand and diminish depending on each person. Human relations training tries to increase the size of Quadrant I, the open area, and reduce the blind and hidden areas. Theorists and trainers who use this model are not sure what to do about the unknown quadrant.

J. Luft thought it was important for individuals to enlarge the "open" aspect of their lives by self-disclosure and to reduce the blind area through soliciting feedback from others. You can see how this might enhance effectiveness in the workplace and in relationships. Greater interpersonal effectiveness is a key goal in successful managing.

Unassisted homebirth decreases the blind and hidden areas between lovers, because birth is one of life's rare moments where both partners enter the unknown area, making known to each other what was previously unknown. Spouses do not know what they are each capable of doing until they experience an intimate birth.

Then comes baby

Few women choose to birth their babies alone, without their partner. Others desire a midwife and many employ a labor coach at their births. Whatever the circumstance, it is important for the father to be fully involved in the pregnancy and birth process since he was very involved in the conception of the child. Both partners conceived the child together and it seems logical they should both embrace birth, the beginning of their parenting journey together.

Traditional birth experiences pull a couple apart rather than strengthen their unity. Hospital delivery leaves the husband in a peripheral role rather than a central one. Midwives may boast of their ability to facilitate satisfying births, but their mere presence places the father in a secondary role, even if he catches his own baby. The midwife's presence conveys to the father that he alone is unfit to be fully and solely ("soul-ly") involved in the birth.

Couples should contemplate how they want to birth their babies and what their goals are for a good birth. Think about what you want out of life. Some are satisfied with the absence of loneliness, fear, pain and suffering. Others stop at mate-rial gratifications. Others seek success and recognition. Many want total fulfillment including love, peace and hap-piness. Attempting to form a special union with your mate is one way to fulfillment, and how you birth your baby will play a major role in marital and life fulfillment.

A couple's unity begins to form with ideas they each bring to the relationship. These ideas contribute to goals so that at the time of their engagement, or commitment to spend a lifetime together, the couple is laying a foundation. Then a special unity takes place on their wedding day, and develops during conception, throughout pregnancy and as they ven-ture through parenthood. Unity is strengthened every time the couple includes each other during major events, especially childbirth. How a couple emerges from pregnancy and child-birth contributes to their relationship, personhood, and par-enthood.

A powerful physical and psychological union is formed between the couple who births a baby together. Birth tran-scends all rational explanation of time. At the moment of complete surrender, many couples feel a sense of eternity together. They just *know* they will be together forever. Past, present and future are linked together and the baby will be a constant reminder of the momentous event.

Anything other than an unassisted homebirth between lovers is detrimental to the unity the couple yearns for. Men and women are very much separated in the birth experience in the hospital. The helpless husband at the side of the bed can hardly bear to watch his wife in pain as each contraction gets stronger. The baby is born, only to be taken away by a staff of workers in their sterile uniforms.

Midwives attending a homebirth also detract from the couple's sacred unity. When the possibility for a greater spousal unity is interfered with, the couple will not reach the depths required for a deepening of their love.

> There is little chance of marriage and sexuality failing if couples are shielded from those forces that would deny the inseparable connection between the unitive and procreative aspects of the conjugal act of birth. (Moran 1997: 165)

Marilyn Moran discusses "complimentarity." She believes that a healthy marital union which results in children *depends* on a birth that involves the husband accepting the baby into his hands. During coitus, he plants the seed, and during birth, he accepts the baby, bringing sexuality to full circle where feminine and masculine qualities merge.

> By engaging in a conjugal dialogue, both members of the love dyad gain access to their own latent faculty character- istic of their mate's experience and to personally display, even if only briefly, that with which the other has been so generously endowed. This means that she who customar- ily receives must become convex and penetrating, for a change, and he, the initial convex penetrator must now try his hand at being concave and receiving. The opportunity for this comes during the conjugal act of birth. (Moran 1997: 42)

Intimate husband and wife birth is a *necessity* for those who desire a deep marital bond. I have come to believe this after accepting the following statements as truths: (1) Birth is a sexual event (2) Sex is something that should be done pri- vately, in a committed loving relationship, preferably mar- riage and (3) If birth is a sexual event, it too should be done in private.

The physiology of birth has been compared to sex by sev- eral authors including Marilyn Moran and Diana Korte, among others. William and Martha Sears describe the simi- larities between birth and sex in *The Birth Book*. (1) The hormone oxytocin, which enhances labor and produces or- gasm, is present during both events. (2) A woman who is comfortable with her sexuality is more likely to surrender during sex and birth.

The birth orgasm

The natural moans and groans of childbirth may be a reflection of pain, but they are also an expression of intense physical activity. The sighs, sweat and throbbing immediately before and after birth can be compared to sex. The mind and body are focused on the final moment. Marilyn Moran tells a humorous story of a couple giving birth in an upstairs apartment. When citizens hear noises and gather around to cheer them on during what they think is a sexual encounter, they are very surprised to hear a baby cry a few minutes later!

Birth is likely to be as painful—or pleasurable—as you think it will be. I had read that orgasm could accompany birth and that some couples make love during labor, before the amniotic sac breaks. I was looking forward to the physical pleasure I thought I would have. Unfortunately, my water broke while I was sleeping. So much for foreplay.

Labor pains lasted less than an hour. As with my hospital births, there was no pain a few seconds before the birth. As the baby emerged, it was physically pleasurable, but mainly emotionally satisfying. I was not physically successful in achieving a birth orgasm as described by other women because a part of me still refused to believe it was possible. I was not disappointed; I did not totally surrender myself. I was preoccupied with tearing. Most women try to get birth over as soon as possible and there I was trying to get everything I could out of it. Pardon my selfishness, but we have so few precious births during our lives.

Love and sex

Men and women break off a part from the whole when they isolate sex from love. Babies born to those who do not

> Love is composed of so many sensations, that something new of it can always be said. —Saint Prosper

love each other is also selfish. Mature relationships are able to combine love and sex into self-sacrifice and servitude.

Picture a young couple in love outwardly expressing their physical attraction, while oblivious to all else in the world. Nothing can penetrate the energy force that surrounds them. Picture them inside an enormous magical bubble. Their first few weeks or months of courtship are spent inside this bubble. As the couple settles into the stress and routine of life and as their relationship matures, their bubble does not seem to be so evident. Yet it is still there and still strong.

Many "bubbles" continue to get stronger. The physical expressions become less obvious. Couples who believe it is their obligation to seek a doctor and have a hospital birth are destroying the bubble that has been shielding them from outside forces. Assembly-line obstetrics may even be the couple's first experience of interference. When more couples realize that they should remain home for birth, they will keep their bubble of love intact, and will discover that it becomes even more impenetrable.

A greater love

Unassisted homebirth can solidify a love relationship, but it will not insulate a couple from future problems or conflicts. Life involves continuous learning and maturing.

Unassisted homebirth leads a couple into a divine dimension of love, complete with trust, dependability and a tenderness which cannot be experienced even during the most beautiful moments of passionate lovemaking. The depth of the couple's love can never be taken away. It is meant to be shared with others, especially the new family. Love continues to intensify, rather than fade, as time goes on, and as partners discover greater treasures in each other.

"Thus it is in the forgetting of self, in a certain anticipation and ready obedience to the needs and desires of the partner that genuine, lasting satisfaction and true sharing and possessing of the beloved are accomplished." (Imbiorski 1969: 86) A couple in love can reach an intense level of physical and emotional serenity during sex, and the couple can reach an even higher level of forgetting themselves during an intimate birth experience. The husband and wife may be focusing on both themselves and each other, but a third party, the baby, is the main focus at birth. This element is not present during sex.

After a couple has gone through an unassisted homebirth, other problems in life seem to pale in comparison. A new facet of the husband's and wife's personalities is discovered, as is a greater sense of awe and respect. The homebirthing couple may even feel like young lovers, whereas parents seldom describe this kind of intensity after a hospital birth. Because the unassisted homebirth strengthens the unity of most couples, it is likely that each partner's selfishness diminishes. This may serve as a deterrent to infidelity and poor communication, which weaken the marital bond.

Men are from Mars, Women are from Venus, by John Gray, spent over five years on the top ten bestsellers list during the 1990's. The popularity of this book and other self-help books aimed at improving relationships shows that men and women are very concerned about understanding each other. If the same people who buy these books knew the phenomenal power of unassisted birth, there would be an explosion in happiness and well-being in many marriages across the country.

Gray described the "seasons of love."

> A relationship is like a garden. If it is to thrive it must be watered regularly. Special care must be given, taking into account the seasons as well as any unpredictable weather. New seeds must be sown and weeds must be pulled. Similarly, to keep the magic of love alive we must understand its seasons and nurture love's special needs. (Gray 1992: 283)

Couples who have gone through unassisted birth and have shared the excitement of springtime or the rewards of autumn are much better equipped to deal with the challenges of summer and winter.

Fusion of personalities

Because there is total privacy between lovers, it is likely that there will be a fusion of personalities during the birth. Having a child is the most creative thing a couple can do. The baby is a permanent example of the joining of the couple's hearts and minds. If the parents share in the process of making and raising the child, they should have a meaningful sharing at the birth event.

Odds are against a couple trying to achieve a fusion where there are others present at the birth or if the setting is even somewhat uncomfortable. Intimate birth is so emotionally appealing that it's easy to lose sight of the physical pain that often accompanies childbirth. No separations between the couple, no small talk or interference from strangers, nobody barking commands at the couple—what a way to have a baby!

While the couple is strengthening their bond during the birth, they are also beginning parenthood with confidence. By seeing each other in a new situation, one that takes courage, a special, mutual respect takes place. If they triumph after a birth experience, they can do anything; they are ready to take on the world.

DIY birth often results in more intimacy and a stronger marriage. Here are some of the responses from the husbands and wives who completed the questionnaire.

How has the DIY changed both of your lives? Do you feel more connected to your mate, your child?

> Yes. Having Bill be my sole partner for the last birth was so special. My trust and appreciation of him deepened.

> Yes. We both feel much more connected to each other and to our DIY birth children and all of our children. We are much more willing and positive about working out all the little and big problems that go along with having a large family and this brings us even closer.

My husband seemed more attached to the DIY child. And so proud! He treated me like a queen. He seemed more sure of himself as a dad.

The DIY birth has given me more confidence, especially in God. My husband feels that he has attained "spiritual completion as headship in the home." We are definitely more bonded to each other. There is a special bond with baby too, though we love all four kids!

Definitely. I feel more connected to my mate, my children, Mother Earth, all women, my mother and grandmother.

I think the fact that my husband is the very first person to touch the babies is a source of pride for him. He caught his children in his own hands. Having our babies at home has caused me to trust my husband more. My life and the lives of our children were totally entrusted to his discernment of the way labor was progressing. I think we are more connected because of our having had our babies at home together.

I believe Peter and I have grown even closer than we were, and we've always had a tight family. The births have also encouraged us to seek God for everything in life, whether big or small. Our two older sons have grown spiritually, knowing that what they prayed for was heard and answered by God. As a family, I believe we will always be closely connected to each other and Christ.

I feel much closer to my husband, more pride, more trust, warmer feelings in general. The DIY has made me proud of myself, too.

Keith Steinke admits, "I feel much closer to Cindy as well. I feel that there was a special event that only Cindy, Celeste, and of course, Corinne took part in."

Yes. We are more trusting of each other to rely on for survival. A greater respect was born from our DIY birth.

Kim Pratt says of her unplanned unassisted homebirth:

It was such a normal, natural seeming thing that it didn't really change us. Both of us agree that we wish we could say it brought us closer, but we were already so close that neither of us feels any different. As far as feeling more connected to our child, I felt really close to my son who was born in a hospital. I think I was more at peace with my homebirth because I wasn't afraid of anyone taking my baby away and doing things I felt like I should be doing, such as bathing, or things I didn't approve of. We were in control.

Falling in love is like springtime. We feel as though we will be happy forever. We cannot imagine not loving our partner. It is a time of innocence. Love seems eternal. It is a magical time when everything seems perfect and works effortlessly. Our partner seems to be the perfect fit. We effortlessly dance together in harmony and rejoice in our good fortune. —John Gray

9

Men And Birth

Irrevocable damage is done to a man when he is prevented from personally receiving his wife's gift of love at the moment of childbirth. When birth is experienced as a genuine husband/wife love encounter, as it was intended to be, dignity and life are restored to a man and a new tomorrow made possible. (Moran 1981: 65)

Birth is not just for women

Women should be and are more involved in their own pregnancies than their husbands. Still, fathers are very much excluded. Men who are involved in the pregnancy, birth, rearing and education of their children contribute to the well-being of the family. Since the man's involvement as a father begins with the birth experience, what better way to cooperate in childrearing than to have an important responsibility in the childbearing act?

Why have women left many fathers sitting on the sidelines while they go off to doctors appointments? Why are women more eager to talk with their girlfriends about "women" stuff and prefer to share their pregnancies and birth with other women rather than their husbands? Why aren't more people best friends with their spouses? By choosing to leave their partners in another dimension when it comes to those "female" times (which are actually "couple" times), they are leaving men out of an important part of their lives. How can fathers be expected to be fully involved if women do not involve them from the onset? Is it that men are bored, do not care, or is it because they have been shut out?

Childrearing is thought of as primarily women's work. Some men choose to be uninvolved in pregnancy, birth, childrearing or abortion decisions. Others are intentionally left out by women. "Traditional" men believe that childrearing begins and ends with their financial support. Modern fathers are choosing to form more meaningful relationships with their children because they know that their children crave an emotional involvement with them.

Many years ago, fathers were not allowed to witness their children's hospital births. Today, a father is expected to physically and emotionally support the mother in the labor room with tasks such as correct breathing, holding her hand, rubbing her back and staying by her side. He may even have the pleasure of cutting the cord. Still, the father is disconnected from the full experience of birth. The father's role in a traditional birth is that of a manager. Although he may not realize it, he is being insulted. When the doctor, staff and hospital policies dictate the birth, the father is assigned a job that pacifies, but does not truly involve him.

Dad is proud of himself for being so involved throughout the pregnancy and birth since he attended all the childbirth classes and was able to help his wife through such an ordeal. He has been socialized to picture the time when men were not allowed in delivery rooms. He has played his "major role" in his wife's delivery and as he emerges from the birthing room, he now feels his life is complete with a new baby. The staff is happy about the father's non-threatening and non-confrontational role. He is kept out of their way and he does not ask any questions. He is unaware of any other role he could have played in the birth event.

> A woman who loves does not fear ridicule; a man in love knows no pride.

Fear and trembling

Some women desire an unattended birth, but their husbands do not. Many couples do not have unassisted births when the fathers are fearful or not interested, but some women may still persist. Refusal to accept his child into his hands at the moment of birth is more likely a result of the father's learned behavior than innate aversion. A forty week gestation period is usually sufficient time for a couple to undo some cultural conditioning and prepare for the birth.

A husband opposed to DIY birth when the mother desired it has resulted in various outcomes: (1) the mother delivers at a hospital (2) the mother has an attendant at home (3) the mother has a DIY birth with a nervous or unprepared husband (4) the mother has a solo birth.

Some men prefer to keep their distance from childbirth because they believe the myths or may be uncomfortable with the responsibility. Catching the baby at home with no medically experienced help can be very intimidating. The masculine preference for control and management are not apparent during a free-flowing birth. Men prefer order and independence, rather than the feminine elements of flexibility, compromise, tenderness, and dependence which are at the forefront of unassisted birth.

Reluctant fathers

Must an unassisted birth be a mutual decision between the partners? That's for you to answer. Couples who generally agree upon how many children they would like and how they will bear and rear them encounter less conflict than couples with opposing values and ideas. It would benefit couples to decide how they will birth a baby before a pregnancy. There is almost no talk of birth choices when couples assume that childbirth automatically takes place in a hospital with a doctor.

Some fathers are fixated on the sight of blood and mucous. They worry about what to do with the placenta, how to cut the cord, or how to alleviate their wife's pain; they are preoccupied with negative thoughts. One way women can ease their husbands fears is to talk, study and plan with them. A calm woman can often convince her husband that everything will be all right for the upcoming birth, and a reluctant father may embrace an unassisted birth if he truly respects his wife and has faith in the process.

No man should be forced to participate in a birth he is opposed to, nor should a pregnant woman make a secret decision to involve him without his consent. These situations create a chance that a stressful birth will follow, along with marital conflicts.

Fully involved

Men of past generations awaited news of their baby's birth in hospital waiting rooms, while today's men think they are being involved in childbirth, but they are actually being shown the birth process. Only unassisted birth enables fathers to fully participate.

Jim Hunt, of Colchester, Connecticut describes his participation in his wife's pregnancy:

> I began to feel even closer to Beth during this time. Our hands-on discoveries entailed touching in new ways and growing sensitivity on my part as to her body's changes. I also felt that I knew the new little person in a very direct and clear way. I began to love the baby inside Beth as our child. I loved Beth more and more each passing week, especially as I understood what she was having to stoically bear to have our baby inside and to birth her. (Moran 1997: 184)

I've spoken to many women who would love to give birth unassisted, but their husbands are scared to death so they end up hiring a midwife or going to the hospital. —Laura Kaplan Shanley

Men who have been the first person to see and touch their babies often develop a new perspective on sex. Because they have partaken in a miraculous event which results from intercourse, sex with their wives often becomes more emotional and spiritual. Those elements may have been present before the unassisted homebirth, but a new significance is attached to sex, much to the wife's contentment.

Any of the men who have assisted their wives in delivery of their babies will tell you that although they may have been uncomfortable with the initial feelings of vulnerability, the growth from the experience far outweighed the emotional risks. In fact, many of the men feel that their lives lacked something, especially if they compare the unassisted homebirth to a hospital birth or dissatisfying midwife-attended delivery.

Many men do not feel they can truly express themselves. What makes a person true to himself is the degree to which he can feel comfortable enough to openly express emotions. When emotions are suppressed, other problems are manifested. A man who births his own baby with his wife in the privacy of their own bedroom is among the very few who will feel a different kind of closeness and connection to his lover and child. If that experience does not bring out the most tender side of a man, I do not know what will. This softer side of masculinity contributes immensely to emotional health and stability of the man and often the marriage. A man's feelings for his lover are intensified as he witnesses her give birth freely, without fear or inhibitions. Unassisted homebirth lays the foundation for greater confidence, achievement and compassion in all areas of life.

Most fathers are meager spectators in the childbearing process rather than responsible participants. In comparing the difference between a hospital birth and a DIY homebirth, I can honestly say that America's approach to birth is exploitative and abusive to couples, both psychologically and physically. Men deserve more respect during birth.

Men's stories

The birth stories which appear towards the end of the book are written by the mothers. Fathers' testimonies appear on the next several pages.

Bob Griesemer

I have put off for a long time writing my comments for Lynn's book. She has the whole thing written now except for my input so I better write this. I guess one of the reasons it's taken so long for me to write my thoughts down about our homebirth is that it was just so awesome that I feel like I can't even come up with words adequate enough to describe it. Let me try anyway.

When Lynn first mentioned the idea of giving birth to our baby at home I told her she was crazy! No way was I going to allow that. I was the man of the house and it was my responsibility to protect and watch out for the well being of the family and I just felt that giving birth at home away from the professional medical support was just plain irresponsible if not downright dangerous. Well, that was because I had bought into the prevailing notion that childbirth is inherently risky and fraught with danger that requires the constant supervision of trained medical people. Little did I know just how wrong that notion was.

Lynn does not give in to me that easily so she worked and worked on me to educate me about the idea of homebirth. I am not too stubborn and will change my mind if I am presented with new information so I did some reading and listened to Lynn with an open mind. It was when I read Marilyn Moran's book *Birth and the Dialogue of Love* that I realized we should have a homebirth.

It was Marilyn who made me realize that birth is part of a couple's love just as conception is. I concluded that I was missing something from our four prior hospital births. I was not a participant; I didn't have a role to play; I was extra. I just stood around trying to talk soothingly to Lynn and holding her hand (when she let me), but the focus of attention was on the medical surroundings and all the interventions, the constant stream of strangers into the room to check on progress, to hook up the fetal monitor, to insert the IV during one of the births. I felt so unneeded one time I went and got myself a sandwich for lunch, leaving Lynn there knowing the medical people would be watching her. I know that seems pretty cold and heartless of me, but I feel that the situation contributed to that. As I recall, it was actually the doctor who suggested I go get some lunch.

Then we got close to delivery (still talking about the other four hospital deliveries) and that's when I really became superfluous. In all four of our hospital births there would come a time during labor when Lynn would not want to hear from me or touch me. At our first birth she told a nurse she wanted to hear her, not me, and wouldn't let me touch her.

At the time I didn't think it bothered me because I'd heard all the jokes about the wife in labor who blames her husband for doing that to her and all that. I think we tell those jokes just so we won't have to seriously think about what's going on around us in that delivery room, because if you stop and think about it, which I've done now thanks to Lynn, you'll realize that in most cases the hospital delivery room is the last place you want to be to have a baby with your wife. Men, you would never let another man between your wife's legs while she's lying in bed half naked in your bedroom, right? Yet you give up that position when she's in the hospital to have a baby and you don't think twice. I think there is something wrong with that.

A baby is born and he is beautiful and wonderful and a miracle from God. In the hospital you have about a minute to contemplate that before the trained medical personnel grab the baby and whisk him off to do whatever their training says they're supposed to do with him. Once again I didn't think there was anything wrong with that because after all, they are highly trained, skilled medical professionals who know what they're doing. Well, that might be true but what they're doing is not necessarily for the good of the baby or the mother. What's best for baby and mom is for them just to be together, to start nursing, but at a minimum to be held close and to look at each other. Don't believe that talk about how newborns can't see. If you were in a dark room for nine months and then were suddenly brought out into a room with bright lights like the average hospital room and then had some eye drops put right in your eyes, you'd probably not see very well either. But, if instead, you were brought out into a room with low lighting and were left alone, like a baby is if born at home, you might see much better.

I thought about those four hospital births and about what I'd read in Marilyn Moran's book about birth really being a dialogue of love between husband and wife and realized that giving birth in the quiet comfort of our own home really would be much better.

The moment of Millicent's birth will be forever etched in my mind as the most significant moment of my life. I can hardly begin to describe the feelings and the emotions of the moment, to see that little purple head start emerging from my wife's body, and then the rest of her just slipping out into my waiting hands. I was the first one in the whole world to hold my baby. What a miracle from God, what a gift from my wife! Time stood still. The rest of the world ceased to exist. All that mattered was the task at hand, assisting Lynn as she labored and catching Millicent as she came into the world. When it was all over and Mom and baby were settled down and comfortable and things were cleared up, I couldn't get back to sleep. I was on an adrenaline rush the whole time. I remember feeling like I just had four or five cups of coffee. It was such an intense experience.

Guys, if you want to gain a whole new appreciation for the miracle of life and for your wife then catch your own baby. You'll also feel more of an attachment to that child too. I feel different about Millicent than my other four that were caught by doctors in the hospital. I don't mean to say I love Millicent any more than Robby, Melanie, Hilary or Christina. I love all my children as unique and special gifts from God entrusted by him to my and Lynn's care, but there is just something there with Millicent that isn't with the others. I really believe she even reacted to my voice differently as an infant, almost as if she knew that I was the first one to hold her. I should have had that with all my children and if I had it to do over again, I would have had all of them at home.

The following are some of my answers to the questions on the questionnaire that Lynn sent out soliciting stories to appear in this book. They give some more of my thoughts that I didn't include in my story above.

Briefly state why you had a DIY homebirth:

I must admit that I originally did not want a homebirth. When my wife first mentioned the idea to me I thought she was nuts, quite literally. She had to work on me for awhile to get me to accept the idea. After having gone through it now I can wholeheartedly say that I'm glad she convinced me. She gave me lots of reading material to help me understand the process. It wasn't until I read Marilyn Moran's book, *Birth and the Dialogue of Love* that I became convinced that a homebirth was the way to go. I think at that point I was convinced of a homebirth but still wanted a midwife present just in case.

Well, we interviewed one midwife but just didn't click. We weren't comfortable enough with her and we didn't really have any other choices so I think that's when the unassisted idea started to gain a hold of us. We decided we would do it ourselves and just ask a couple friends of ours over to help out with the children. One friend is a registered nurse and the other is studying to be a midwife so we felt like that was good expertise to have around. We got a copy of *Emergency Childbirth* by Dr. Gregory White and I read through that. I think between that book and Marilyn Moran's book, I was definitely convinced that we could do this ourselves. I was especially impressed by *Emergency Childbirth* when it ended one chapter by saying that any reasonably intelligent eight year-old could do it. When I thought about it, I realized that they don't have any books called "Emergency Appendectomies" or "Emergency Brain Surgery" for laymen to use if they should just happen to find themselves in that situation, yet they have one on childbirth that anyone can use. It really made me wonder why we had allowed highly paid obstetricians to deliver our other four children while I stood by watching. All four turned out to be textbook pregnancies and from what we've read, 80 to 90% of deliveries do not need qualified medical intervention.

How was your frame of mind regarding fear, anxiety, tension during the pregnancy? How did you prepare to deal with fear?

My frame of mind as the father was actually based on Lynn's frame of mind. She's the one that goes through it directly and she had done it four times before so she felt very confident and so, I felt confident. My religious faith helped tremendously. No matter how humans try to control the process of life with artificial means of contraception and abortion, there is still that unknown, unexplainable element. It is truly a miracle the way new life enters the world and it definitely is evidence of a higher being controlling it all. To have a belief in God provided the source of strength we needed to deal with this most natural of conditions that God provides for us for the procreation of the race.

What are some techniques, strategies or practices you can share that helped you have a smooth delivery?

You need to prepare beforehand and have everything ready to go. We had prepared some homemade containers made out of rolled up newspaper surrounded by plastic to catch the afterbirth and fluids. We also had big plastic sheets we were able to lay down between the bed and the bathroom door to help keep things clean. We also had a plastic sheet down on the bed under the regular sheets. That all removed the worry about messing things up and helped me concentrate on the task at hand which was assisting Lynn in giving birth.

We ordered a homebirth kit which had all the medical supplies like plastic gloves, sterile pads and umbilical cord clamps that they use in the hospital. I didn't bother with the gloves but the cord clamps were handy. Just having everything ready helped make it a smooth birth.

Did you experience any fear, anxiety or tension during the birth?

I did not experience any fear or anxiety. We had done a lot of reading and were pretty much prepared for just about anything and had done a lot of praying and really felt God's presence. I remember having this sense that this is the right thing to do and that God was right there with us helping out, comforting me throughout the whole thing because I really didn't think about it. It was amazing, that's all I can say. I never felt so fully human, so fully alive before in my life. Lynn was a psychology major in college and I would always kid her about her "touchy, feely" theories that she studied, but after our homebirth, she happened to read aloud to me the following passage:

> In such states of **peak experience**, we experience phenomena in their simplicity, 'oughtness', beauty, goodness, and completeness. There is a lack of strain, an effortlessness, a spontaneity about the experience that is almost overwhelming. Typically there is a lack of consciousness of space and time. Intense emotions such as wonder, awe, and reverence are felt. During these intense experiences, individuals transcend their own selfishness. Events and objects are perceived as they truly are and are not distorted to meet the experiencers' needs or wishes. (Ryckman 1982: 370)

I thought she was reading something out of a book describing homebirth, but it was from one of her psychology textbooks discussing Abraham Maslow's hierarchy of needs; in particular, the highest state of self-actualization. That passage on peak experiences describes our homebirth experience exactly. It was astounding.

How did the emotional experience compare to other births?

This one was much different. I was always impressed with each of our other four births in the hospital. I saw them as miracles from God regardless of where they took place, but I always felt like there was something missing deep in the back of my mind after all of them. After Millicent's birth, I realized that what was missing was my involvement. What a difference it made.

What would I do differently next time?

We would stay away from the doctor's office more. We'd probably make one visit in order to obtain a doctor's signature certifying that Lynn was pregnant so that the State could provide the birth certificate. We would also be honest and forthcoming with the doctor to avoid any misunderstandings and/or resentments. Lynn's doctor would not release her records and wanted to charge $50.00 just for a letter saying she was pregnant. We finally asked our primary care physician to do the letter and she agreed.

Give a few adjectives to describe three months postpartum.

This time was much less stressful due to having the baby at home. It was just the family and it was nice. We even had a birthday party for Millicent the day she was born. Of course she didn't get much out of it, but we had fun! Lynn baked cupcakes and we had a little party and gave the other kids gifts to celebrate all around. It was great. We kept Millicent away from the well-baby pediatric visits and that greatly reduced the stress level. I think well-baby visits is an oxymoron. If you're well, you don't need a doctor.

My experience with my co-workers after the birth was very different compared to my other children's births. When I called our secretary to tell her the good news, I said Millicent had been born at home but didn't say whether we planned it or whether it was an emergency or what. Well, I found out when I got back to work that many of them had speculated as to whether we had planned it or whether it just happened too suddenly for us to get to the hospital in time. There was almost an office pool going to bet on which way it was. I was sort of a celebrity for awhile when I returned. They started calling me "Doctor Bob." I think almost everyone was impressed with what we had done.

How has the DIY birth changed both of our lives? Do we feel more connected to our mate/child?

I think it's definitely brought us closer together as a couple. We each have a better appreciation for each other. I have a much greater respect for Lynn as a woman after uniting with her in this birth. I'm even more amazed at the whole process of pregnancy and birth now. I definitely feel more connected to both Lynn and our children. Even though we had the other four children in hospitals, I think having the last one at home has given me a closer connection to all my children and definitely with Millicent. She seemed to be very relaxed in my arms from the very beginning. There were times with all of our children when I just couldn't quiet or comfort them and would have to hand them over to Mom.

With Millicent, there were very few times when I had to do that. She would be making noise as an infant and I would walk into the room and say something and she would immediately quiet down and start listening. It was amazing. I think that because I was the first one she came in contact with in this world, there will always be a special connection. Every father should have that kind of connection with his children. This doesn't in any way diminish the mother's role, of course, since it is she who carries the child for nine months and can breastfeed the child, but what it does do is increase the father's role and make it more significant.

Any other suggestions or comments?

FATHERS, CATCH YOUR BABIES! You will find a closer attachment to your family than you had before and a better appreciation of them. I think that the unassisted homebirth method is best so that husband and wife can be as intimate as they were when the child was conceived. If you feel you need an attendant there, be it a midwife or a doctor in a hospital, insist that you be allowed to catch your baby. You won't be sorry.

Matt Bunkelman

Believe it or not, I was more afraid for Wendy with our second pregnancy than I was with our first. Since we experienced pre-term labor more than once with our first, I was afraid that it would happen again. Although I can't explain it, my fear was eased when we decided to have a midwife-attended homebirth.

I was experiencing anxiety over the typical male bread-winner concerns such as insurance, another mouth to feed (at least after breastfeeding was no longer the staple source of nourishment), and other financial concerns. I became even more anxious about the financial concerns after I found out that the homebirth would have to be paid for up front.

I had just started a new job with excellent benefits and Wendy had a hard time convincing me that the homebirth was the best thing for us. I guess that I was thinking too much like a modern man and not listening to what my wife and my heart was saying to do. The fear was easiest to cope with since immediately after we discovered the pregnancy, we contacted the certified nurse midwives that delivered our first. We believed that this pregnancy would be better managed with hindsight as a factor even after we decided on the homebirth. The anxiety would always be there, just easier to suppress.

I didn't have time to experience any fear, anxiety or tension during the birth. I can replay the events surrounding the day Abigail Li was born more vividly than any other day in my twenty-eight years. No single event in my life was more tantamount than that day, and I'm sure that none will ever compare.

Thanks to modern technology, I felt a vibration at my hip that sent an immediate shiver up my spine. I was at work, and as circumstances would have it, this was the only day of the week I was slated to be in earlier than my scheduled time. It was about two weeks before Wendy's due date, but something told me that the page I was receiving was the one I was waiting for. After a brief telephone conversation with Wendy, I told my supervisor that the time had come. I ran the whole way to my car even though the steel processing plant where I work is over a city block long.

I believe I set a new record for traveling from Detroit to Monroe. I even stopped along the way to ask a Michigan State police officer for assistance, but he was too busy writing a ticket and told me simply to be careful. I made a forty-five minute drive in twenty-five minutes with top speeds somewhere around 110 miles per hour. I didn't really notice though; I was more concerned about making it home in time.

When I pulled into the drive, I ran into the house and saw that my mother was there to take Carly, our firstborn, home with her. I didn't even notice that the midwives had not arrived. My mother told me that Wendy was in the bathroom, but she didn't have time to finish her sentence when I heard Wendy call out to me and moan. My heart was racing faster than I was driving down I-275 just minutes ago, but I collected my thoughts and headed for the bathroom.

As I walked down the hall, it hit me that the midwives hadn't arrived yet. I went into the bathroom more terrified than I had ever been, but I knew I had to be as cool as Bogey so Wendy wouldn't sense anything and panic. The bath was running and Wendy looked scared, yet so beautiful. I smiled at her and searched for the right thing to say, but simply blurted out, "Is everything okay?" If looks could kill, I don't know who would have delivered the baby.

Wendy was concerned that our midwives hadn't gotten there yet, and something about not being able to make breakfast for Carly and do the dishes before my mother got there. I laughed and started washing my hands with scalding hot water, not noticing my skin melting. Thank God Wendy started telling me what to do or I would have been over the sink washing my hands like Lady Macbeth while Wendy gave birth. She told me to get the sheets on the bed and set out the supplies from our homebirth kit. I ran into the bedroom only to run right back into the bathroom as Wendy was hit with a powerful contraction.

I rubbed her back as she was on all fours in the tub and did my best to talk her through. When the pain subsided, I returned to the bedroom only to be called back into the bathroom. This went on for about five minutes before I realized that the contractions were only minutes apart and getting closer and closer together. I was so consumed with what I was trying to do that I didn't have time to think about what was happening.

By this time, I was certain that the midwives weren't going to make it and we were on our own. I tried my best to keep Wendy's mind off this, but I think my mother felt it out in the living room. It was here, that time stopped; Wendy and I became the only two beings existing on the Earth. I was afraid to look between Wendy's legs, but when I did, I saw her vagina swollen and pulsating and I knew what was about to happen. I told myself to take a deep breath and try to remember everything we learned in our classes. The hand of God was definitely on us and I felt as though I was outside of myself looking over my shoulder at a man and a woman doing what was intended since Life began.

Wendy moaned one more time and I saw her vagina expand as the head crowned. I told her that I could see the head and she should take a deep breath before she pushed. As the head came out, her water broke and I was so focused on what was happening that I wasn't even phased by it. As Abigail turned her head up toward me I found myself staring into the most beautiful pair of blue-in-blue eyes I had ever seen.

At that moment I realized that I would never again experience an event more sublime and life-affirming than being the first person Abigail would see and feel.

I told Wendy that the head was out and everything was all right, and she could push when she was ready. I thought of my father (who passed away many years ago) and the first football pass he ever threw to me as I remembered the advice of our childbirth educator; "catching a baby is like catching a football." I knew that he was right there over my shoulder as I caught the most important "pass" ever. Wendy just had to push once and Abigail slid out onto my left arm as I brought my right hand up to cradle her lithe body. I felt the electricity of life course through me straight into my soul.

I announced to Wendy that it was a girl and I think the three of us started to cry. Wendy was the first to remember that the first few minutes after birth are the most critical and brought us back to reality. I asked her what to do and we both were a little confused, but decided that we should head into the bedroom. The only question in my mind was, "How?" Wendy suggested that I hand Abigail to her between her legs and she would walk to the bed. I did just that and Wendy proved to me, not for the first time, that Woman is the most awesome of all God's creatures as she strolled into the bedroom with a newborn in her arms and an umbilical cord dangling between her legs. I think it took me a few minutes to collect myself after seeing her do that after having just given birth.

We were both so flustered but relieved as we tried to remember what to do next. I went to turn up the thermostat as Wendy put the bonnet on Abigail and bundled her up. I totally forgot that my daughter and mother were in the other room and I told them we had a baby girl in the bedroom. As they went back into the bedroom to see, I noticed the first midwife's van pulling up outside. At this moment I almost swooned as the gravity of what had just transpired washed over me like a wave. I collected myself, greeted the midwife at the door, and told her, "Come on in. It's too bad you missed all the fun!"

Frank Pratt

Although we planned on a midwife attended homebirth, I voraciously read everyday, to be fully ready for each and every problem that could arise. I would read about other births and determine my course of action for each situation. If a mind is allowed to wallow in fear and anxiety, then it cannot function properly. Knowing this, I have tried to keep myself as calm and collected as I could. Little did I know that our midwife would be a "no-show" and I would be called upon to undertake a tremendous responsibility.

Having gone past the due date was a blessing, for it allowed me more time to prepare for the birth. The incompetent cervix that my wife was supposed to have certainly seemed to be competent. Knowing that we made it past term was a good sign that the baby would be of a healthy weight and have fully developed lungs.

The day of the birth was a glorious June day. My day started with my usual routine of going to work, ensuring that my beeper was in working condition. I had been carrying it with me for the length of our pregnancy. At times, it seemed that my hip was vibrating even when the beeper wasn't activated. On this day, it would be the tingling sensation I was anticipating. Although it was not the emergency code we had selected, I still raced to the phone knowing that this was "it." Kim told me she had taken the castor oil and that she didn't feel very good. I left work and hurried home.

When I arrived home, my wife was in a frustrated state because the castor oil not only tasted bad, but caused discomfort. I was glad to be home to help and with Kim close to the bathroom, I took our two year old son, Gannon outside to play. A little later, my wife suggested we go for a walk in the park.

We had a nice time at the park, walking and relaxing. Kim seemed to be introspective and off by herself. As Gannon and I were throwing stones in the bay, Kim said nothing was wrong, but that maybe we should go home. On the way home, we bought some incredible sunflowers to transplant, restocked our food supply and settled in at home. Kim told me she was too tired to do anything, so she took a nap while Gannon and I played some more.

I was in the backyard when I heard her yell. Kim's water had broken during her nap and she was definitely in labor. She took charge and told me to clean the bathroom while she made the bed. When I checked on Kim, I found her in the middle of a deep contraction. This worried me slightly because when I called the midwife a few minutes ago, I didn't indicate the need to come over quickly. She lived almost an hour away and I immediately wished I told her to "step on it, and hurry!"

Kim stood up from her contraction, took a deep breath, and continued her task. I was watching her in awe. After another contraction, I told her that I could feel the power coming from her and a growl deep within me led to me believe she was well into second stage labor. We moved to the bathroom where she sat on the toilet and felt like pushing. "No, no," I pleaded, let's go to the bed where I can check to see our progress. When I first glimpsed, I was amazed at what I found—a beautiful little crown of our baby's head was right there, ready to enter the world.

I told Kim it's just you and me. Gannon was pounding at the back door, asking if Mommy was okay. We didn't even have time to let him in. She leaned back against the headboard and let me and Alana take over. As I'm telling Kim to push, I noticed that there was not as much liquid as when Gannon was born and that my timing was off. She was between contractions and I'm praising our creator to let this all work out well. I turned the baby so that her shoulders were sideways and reached under the baby's left armpit and slowly rotated her. That seemed to work and I had the olive oil nearby because I was concerned that Kim would rip in too many places.

One more contraction and out came Alana. I pulled her all the way out and placed her on her mother's breast. What a beautiful sight! Alana was so calm and relaxed and I wish I was too. Mother and baby were bonding as I was running around wondering where the midwife was.

During the birth, I knew just what to do. After I placed her on her mother's breast, I stood back from the scene as if I really wasn't a part of it. I cleared Alana's airways and then I think the intellectual side of my brain, or as some people call it, the left side, proceeded to analyze the input. It was then that fear began to grip my thoughts. "Where was the midwife? Why was Alana so blue? When was the proper time to cut the cord? Why wasn't Alana crying? Why was she so lethargic?" I knew the answers to these questions, but fear drove those to the recesses of my mind. Rather than fully experiencing the splendor of this joyous moment, all I could think about was where the midwife was.

Troy McNear

One year after Ross' birth, my wife Shannon and I were reminiscing about our unassisted homebirth. We were driving on the highway to go Christmas shopping and here's a brief dialogue:

SHANNON: So, what *did* you think of Ross' birth?

TROY: What do you mean?

SHANNON: Well, how was it special to you? Was it special?

TROY: Aaaah! She's got me trapped and now she's going to make me talk! Yes, it was special. It was the most wonderful, fantastic, marvelous experience of my life, getting to deliver my own baby. It's really something when you take complete spiritual headship or responsibility for your family and deliver your own baby. The Lord has blessed us so much. I have a wonderful wife and four beautiful children. For the first time, I'm happy with our finances and where we live. That wasn't always the case, but now I'm satisfied with my life.

SHANNON: What about our relationship? How do you think the homebirth changed it?

TROY: I saw your heart truly turned toward me for the first time. Your attitude did a complete 180 degree turn.

SHANNON: Yes, I feel closer to you too. But isn't it interesting how we each feel that the change was in the other person rather than in ourselves.

Bill Haas

I became convinced that a homebirth was just what I needed after our third child was born in a local hospital. There was such a lack of privacy and so much medical intervention; way beyond what was really necessary.

I don't remember having any real fear or anxiety during Jeanie's pregnancy. If I did, I would always try to deal with it immediately by talking with Jeanie about the concerns, by reading the Bible, and concentrating on key scriptures that we had both been reading previously.

Having babies born here at home has become such a peaceful, comfortable way to have children; not just for me and my wife, but also for our other children as well. Sarah, my oldest was able to help me and be a "go-fer." The others bring their own individual joy and excitement to the new baby just as soon as they are given the chance.

Timing always seems to be a key issue in the birth of a child. As a busy husband, father and worker, having my child born at home is like "having my cake and eating it too." After labor begins and my wife ceases her normal daily routine of being a mom, wife and homemaker, I can still continue to be a dad and worker, while attending to my wife as a husband. So instead of running back and forth to the hospital, I can find myself peacefully placed at home, picking up where my wife left off and still carrying on in a degree of efficiency with work. The birthing atmosphere is very peaceful for me. I feel relaxed, unhurried and very confident that life in my home is in control and under the control of God.

Homebirthing presented a unique opportunity for Jeanie and me to spend time working together, alone without outside interruptions. We would find ourselves working toward a common goal. It was a unique time of bonding, supporting one another, loving and encouraging each other. We became close friends again, and for the first time in some ways. We would occasionally see each other in a new light which only deepened our relationship.

Looking back at our last two homebirths, I can honestly say there were times filled with excitement and joy. They were also times where I found myself growing closer and closer to God. Time and again I would be reading the Bible to myself or maybe out loud to Jeanie and the children. The word is such a deliverer of peace: for Jeanie, in the final stages of labor; the children, when they become anxious; and for myself, for confidence, endurance or communion with my Father.

Until you've delivered at home, it's somewhat difficult to explain how you feel and how exactly it changes you. I know that I would never go back to the old way. And my respect for God's incredible power and authority multiplies one hundred-fold during each birth.

Keith Steinke

When my wife Cindy and I decided to have a homebirth, I felt a little hesitant. The reason I was hesitant is that I'm no doctor. I'm not even in the medical profession. Well, let me tell you, you don't have to be! Cindy got me reading all of the birth books and manuals. Although I did not read all of the books Cindy wanted me to, I read more than she thought. The reading helped me in the end because several things occurred that I had read about. We took a first aid/ CPR course and we notified the local rescue squad of our intentions.

For the last 45 days of the pregnancy, I became increasingly nervous about the birth of our second child. Would I be able to do this? What if she tears? What if the cord is wrapped around the neck? What if...What if...Well, if the world was full of 'what ifs,' we would never get anywhere.

The night Cindy went into active labor was a night like any other. She had about three weeks of pre-labor. Our two year old daughter, Celeste, went to bed around 11:30 P.M. and I went shortly after. Cindy woke me at 12:30 A.M. and told me labor had started. When the big moment arrived, I expected to be nervous and jittery, saying, "What do I do?" Surprisingly, I was dead calm. All of my anxieties were for naught. We set up our birth area and materials, talked a little, then went back and lay down. Cindy got up and got in the tub. Suddenly, Cindy said she was ready, but we were unsure because we were having a hard time checking dilation. Cindy decided to get in the tub and suddenly the baby's head was there. We were able to get Cindy to the birth area and into a squatting position. As she did this, our daughter's head crowned. As her head came out, I noticed that the cord was wrapped twice around the neck. I told Cindy to stop pushing and she said, "I can't." I was able to unloop the cord both times. Then with a plop, Corinne was out. We lifted her up and placed her on Cindy's belly.

We originally planned on having my sister and Cindy's brother at the birth. The more we talked about it, the more we decided against it. The only other witness at Corinne's birth was Celeste. We woke her up around 5:00 A.M. because we wanted her to witness the birth. With her watching the birth I believe it formed a special bond between her and her little sister.

What I felt when Corinne was born is too wonderful to explain. I felt the same way when Celeste was born. It was just a great joy and wonderful feeling to see something you created be born. To other fathers considering this type of birth, I'd say," If you feel confident, go for it." I really liked not having anyone else there and I think it helps the family bonding to be alone. I plan on doing this again for the next baby!

Michael Scimeca

There really is something to this homebirth thing but it is not for everyone. It has to be something that people inherently *know* they have to do and not just something they *want* to do.

Before we knew that we were having our first child, my wife Allison and I decided we wanted to have a homebirth. When she suggested that I too be naked during the labor, I knew right then that there would be no midwife. Fortunately, we share the same philosophy of honoring the life force. Having a homebirth was never debated.

Our birth was to be a very intimate and sacred event. To prepare for this we packed lunch which included warm water, grape juice, raisins, plums and bananas. We had a crockpot on hand so that I was able to keep applying heat to her perineum which she instinctively wanted. We spread newspapers throughout our house in order to not confine ourselves to any one specific room. It was our understanding that freedom to move about wherever Allison felt she wanted to be at any given time was an important accommodation. This showed itself to be true when toward the end of our labor Allison had an impulsive "urge" to stand in our bathtub at which time she immediately and conveniently broke her water.

The most important job I had was supporting my wife by letting her know how beautiful she was and how wonderful everything was going. During the contractions, which were never more than five minutes apart, I applied heat to her perineum, performed the perennial massage and encouraged her to breathe and not to push. Her main request was that while I performed my duties that I look her straight in the eyes. It was also my job between contractions to make sure that she moved around and had enough fluids on hand to drink.

The theme of our birth which we vocally affirmed throughout was "unconditional faith." At one point I walked into the bathroom and observed Allison with one foot on the bathtub and the other foot on the toilet bowl hanging onto the shower curtain rod and singing. I knew this to be a most unusual occurrence for a childbirth and could do nothing but join her in song. As strange as this sounds, it was a lot of fun. Many times Allison and I kissed and caressed each other. This was without a doubt the most romantic and sexiest moment we had ever shared!

We did not videotape this event which probably added to the intimacy we shared. We had candles burning during the evening to provide our only source of light. We had previously selected music to play softly in the background. I put a "do not disturb" sign on our front door and periodically changed the message on the answering machine to update those concerned friends and family members who were calling. We turned the ringer of our phone off and never knew when a call was coming in. This was our moment! We believe having such reverence for the process of childbirth was the main factor as to why Allison and I had such a pleasurable experience.

We do not believe that it was a coincidence that our wedding song was playing when our baby's head popped out into the world. Five minutes later, my new son and I had our first game of catch. I caught him! It was instantaneous and he seemed to "shoot out" after the shoulders were delivered. The placenta was delivered eleven minutes later at which point my wife let out a big "sigh" seeing that she was no longer physically connected to her baby that she had carried around and bonded with for nine months. It was then that I realized that it would be best for her to cut the umbilical cord. She did so about an hour later. It was appropriate and very symbolic. According to the clock, it was a 30 hour labor.

To this day, Allison and I are certain that it was the fastest 30 hours we had ever spent. Having a homebirth was the only way for us to go. Our son is now two years old and very healthy. He is our pride and joy and is still living on his mother's milk. To say that this experience strengthened our marriage is an understatement. I believe that if people found it in their hearts to have a homebirth, there would be less divorce, less child abuse and it would be a positive step toward world peace. To deny families their right of experiencing this once in a lifetime event is sure to have an effect on everyone involved.

If you can truly come from a place based not on fear, but make an educated and informed choice which honors your belief system, then the end result can be nothing less than the miracle that childbirth is. We are looking forward to having many more unassisted homebirths in the future.

Rick Kohl

My first experience with childbirth was in 1975, with the birth of our eldest daughter, Regina. I was excited and couldn't wait to see and hold my own child; she would get the best start in life and get the best that modern medicine had to offer. Regina was born just like everyone else—in the hospital!

March 28, 1975 finally arrived. We went to the hospital but there wasn't a soul who cared that my wife was in labor. When we finally got to the delivery room, it was all hustle and bustle, bright lights and sterile. The ever-present IV stood there with its needle stuck in Patty's hand. I heard the doctor say to push, but Patty didn't want to push so he pushed her stomach. You can imagine how that felt during a contraction! I heard the snip of scissors for the episiotomy, then, "Here it comes!"

The cord was cut immediately. The doctor held Regina up in mid-air; it was bright and cold and she felt no security around her. Her little arms and legs were stretched out as if in fear. The nurse took her and wiped her off with a rough, sterile cloth. In went the silver nitrate, on went the sterile blanket, and our baby was gone—they just took her away from us! After this, I heard Patty say to me, "NEVER AGAIN IN A HOSPITAL!"

Our next four children were born at home with midwives. Everything was much calmer and pleasant, which enhanced our excitement. After each baby was born, they were wrapped in a soft, warm blanket, placed in their mother's waiting arms, and allowed to nurse. Everything took place in the comfort of our own home. No bright lights and no loud noises. There was no one around who didn't care for or love the new arrival.

When Patty first presented me with the idea of a DIY birth, I was a bit taken aback. I told her I'd have to think about it first. The only midwife we found was similar to a doctor. Home delivery with a midwife is not legal in New York State. (I wonder who came up with that law!?) So, I gave my wife the only logical answer I could. I have to confess that I let my wife take care of most of the details, such as supplies. I think I did this because I was scared. Every other time there was always someone else there to help and give support, but now there would be only myself, my wife, and most likely our eldest daughter who would act as assistant. It was ironic that our first hospital-born child would be assisting at the birth of our first DIY-born child.

About a month before Timothy (our first DIY) was born, I started reading accounts of births from other DIYs to gather strength and courage to do what my wife and I were planning. July 22, 1992 arrived. Patty told us that her water had broken. All fears and inhibitions were set aside; now it was time to get down to the business at hand. As usual, I was tense during the whole labor because of what Patty was going through. Except for my love and support, there was nothing I could do to make it easier for her.

The labor progressed well. Patty was getting tired and I remember thinking, "How can she sleep now?" She fell asleep once and I woke her and told her not to stop now. When Patty got to transition, I remember trying to get her to move closer to the edge of the couch because the thought that was going through my mind was that the angle was too sharp in the birth canal for the baby to make the turn since Patty was sitting up straight. Some of the dumb things that go through your mind are unbelievable!

I have attended the births of all my other children, but never from the position in which I now found myself. When I saw Timothy's head crown, I felt a bolt of electrical excitement go right up my spine. A moment later, I caught our son. I saw my wife give a big smile; her face was just radiating with pleasure. The cord was wrapped around his neck twice. I was scared because it was tight and Patty put me at ease by saying, "Relax." Regina unwrapped it since I was holding Timmy, who was quite slippery. I handed the baby to his mother and he nursed a little right away.

Our second DIY birth went much the same as the first. September 18, 1996 was a calm, pleasant day. Our little girl, Pauline, was born healthy and bright. Since my wife and I are in our 40's, she is definitely a blessing sent from heaven. Over the years I have heard people say that mother and baby bonding is very important, but dad is always left out of this bonding. I have learned from these DIYs that father-baby bonding is just as important. These last two children are special to me because I played a big part in bringing them into the world.

Childbirth is a great gift from our Lord. There is no greater show of love and affection that two people can give to each other than at their child's birth. This gift should not be shared with others outside the family unit.

Would I do a DIY again? Absolutely! If I knew 22 years ago what I know today, all of our children would have been DIY births.

Most of the people we know think we are crazy, but they can't be blamed for their ignorance and the modern propaganda that says only a doctor can give you a healthy baby. They have simply forgotten about the author of life, our Lord and God, Jesus Christ. We only need to put our faith and trust in Him and His most blessed Mother. What could go wrong? What should we fear?

Ad Majorem Dei Gloriam (All for the greater glory of God).

Jesse Wimberley

(from a taped conversation between Jesse and his wife Kirstina)

JESSE: With Cody's birth, the main thing I remember is when he started crowning, I was totally unprepared, and I panicked. I had a real sense of panic and lost my breath. When I realized that it was just the two of us there and it was happening totally in a way that I thought it wouldn't happen and what I mean by that is there was no sign of impending labor. I think the main thing I was feeling is that I wasn't ready. There were supposed to be signs like the water breaking and mucous blood. A sense of calmness came over me when he actually started being born and I saw his face. It all seemed to make total sense. It was a quick transition of just letting go of control and wanting to know what was going on and just kind of accepting that he and you were fine and you all knew what you were doing. I had a very minor role of just catching him.

KIRSTINA: When do you remember labor starting for you?

JESSE: I didn't know. It must have started about 4:00 A.M. and we were asleep. When I woke up, of course, I didn't want to be awake anyway. But spending a year studying the signs of what labor was supposed to look like, in my mind I was going "Well, this is just starting now, we have a long time. It's hours; the best thing to do now is to go back to sleep." So I really wanted the birth to progress the way I in my mind had prepared for it by reading stories about how long it would take (from Spiritual Midwifery, Heart and Hands and Special Delivery). I wasn't prepared at all for it moving that fast. He was born at 6:15 A.M. and it was only a two-hour labor for me.

KIRSTINA: Labor started for me a few hours earlier and I was in the kitchen. Do you remember what you told me when I said I was in labor and to get up?

JESSE: That you should go back to sleep.

KIRSTINA: Because of what?

JESSE: That you should rest until it progresses, that this was the early stages of labor.

KIRSTINA: I told you it wasn't and that I was in full labor and I needed your help.

JESSE: And I tried to time the contractions, but I couldn't time them because you were already so far into labor. You were actually in transition when I even started trying to take you seriously. I was just trying to figure out how far apart they were. They were so close together. And that's when I really panicked, when I realized that there wasn't going to be this long progression of them getting closer and closer, that they were already there. It was past even timing anymore.

KIRSTINA: So you would have time for what?

JESSE: To prepare. To get into what was happening and then I got very nervous when you went into transition and you said, "Take me to the hospital." That was very, very scary.

KIRSTINA: Of course. That's what I always say in transition.

JESSE: The only thing I could think of was, "She must be in transition." That's the only thing I could focus on and that you really didn't need to go to the hospital and you weren't going to die. Then you started doing that kind of birth song and that was very calming to me. I remember that helped a lot because it didn't sound painful; it didn't sound screaming in any way. It was definitely more of a wailing.

KIRSTINA: Let's describe your feelings—panic and all. You couldn't compare it to a hospital birth because you never had one.

JESSE: I lost my breath. I remember not being able to breathe when I first saw that the birth was in process.

KIRSTINA: And do you feel good about wanting to have had a homebirth?

JESSE: Oh yeah! I was the first thing that Cody saw when he came out. He looked at me and we looked at each other. He was very clear in telling me that everything was all right. It was an intense situation to have him look at me and tell me everything was fine. I just needed to catch him.

KIRSTINA: How did this change your life?

JESSE: Well, it changed it in that I feel very much a part of Cody's coming to be, that it wasn't just a woman's situation. It wasn't done away from me and I had a very important role in bringing him into this world. It has set up a dynamic where I could be very close to him on a lot of issues, everything besides breastfeeding It made it much easier for me to be closer in his nurturing and care-giving and just helping him.

KIRSTINA: Where did that put you in place as a man in this world—to have been the only one there instead of some bystander and some other man delivering your child?

JESSE: Well, that's what I'm talking about. It made me feel that I had a much larger role in his being, that birthing wasn't just a woman's situation and a medical situation. I was an integral part of his birth. It's allowed me to not have distance from him in a lot of other stuff since then because it got set up in a way where I was very close to his coming in, so it's made me much closer to him.

KIRSTINA: So it's changed your life by making you feel more a part of childrearing.

JESSE: And often believing that there are things as monumental as birth that are very natural and that having control of the situation is not what was called for. It's a good teaching for me about letting go of control. Cody's birth was also special for me because he was born in the room where his grandmother was born and his great grandfather on my side was born. He was born in the house that his great-grandparents built. He is fourth generation to be in this house. I could feel all the spirits in the room with us. Fifteen minutes after he was born, the sun was coming up and I took him out into the yard to hear the birds who were just waking up. It was a wonderful fall morning. Later on in the day, I took him down to the creek on the farm and baptized him. It was just a wonderful all around day to have here on the farm, starting out with his birth because it's such a continuation of a life-giving process that's gone on here in my family for so many generations.

KIRSTINA: Did you want to have a homebirth?

JESSE: I had never even thought of a homebirth until you said it was something that was important to you. I never even thought about birth in a hospital, at home, or on any level, so it was all new thinking to me. I guess there was some nervousness about a homebirth, thinking that it was a medical process. I started to look at statistics and found that 95% of people presently living on this planet were born at home. Then I had the experience of living in West Africa and seeing all the children born there. Doing the work I do, I am able to question what appears to be the way things normally flow, and birth is certainly the best example I can think of. Learning that birth was not a medical situation was the breakthrough for me of being able to be self-confident enough to be present for that and not worrying what might be wrong.

KIRSTINA: How has the unassisted birth changed our relationship?

JESSE: I see it as a wonderful gift that you gave to me sharing the birth. It's something that we are capable of doing and we don't need to give that power to somebody else. That was a wonderful affirmation for me, that I can deliver babies. When I talk to other men who say, "Oh, I don't know about changing diapers or I don't know about this." If you can deliver a baby, everything else is a piece of cake. Changing diapers, being there when they get hurt, being there when they get sick and being open and understanding is much easier if you're there for that beginning. I think it's very crucial for men that when we get separated out of the birth process, it sets up a dynamic to where that continues throughout the rest of the relationship between the father and that child that they were removed from that. It minimalizes the male experience to have a hospital birth where we are excluded. Being an integral part from the very beginning sets up a dynamic where it's much easier to be a very, very close partner in childrearing forever.

KIRSTINA: Would you have another DIY homebirth?

JESSE: Oh yeah. And we have. The only negative from having the homebirth has been men's reactions. Some men thought my actions were irresponsible. If anything would have gone wrong, it would have been my fault. I believed it for a while and had to get past guilt feelings of "What if something went wrong?" But we decided that if anything went wrong, the hospital was only five minutes away. We talked with midwives and did a lot of reading, talked with men and women about their childbirths.

Scott Gregson

Howdy. My wife twisted my right arm and my left leg to get me to write this. I will do the best that I can. I have been very busy over the years that our four DIY homebirths have occurred, and therefore don't recall all the details and feelings.

When we decided on homebirth for the first time, I believed that God was leading us in that direction. We were both tired of the medical mumbo-jumbo that is pushed upon everybody who walks in the door of a doctor's office. We were not insured. We were broke.

I had been thinking that we could have the birth at home. I reasoned that birth was a natural event, and that it had been done without the help of a doctor at least one or two times before. I had not talked with Charity about my musings.

One day we were talking concerning the baby and the idea was discussed. As it turned out, Charity had been thinking about doing it at home too. We agreed to search the matter out, and Charity went after the data like a pit bull on the tail of a squirrel.

My major concerns were: (1) Charity's health and safety, (2) the baby's well-being, because we could do nothing but watch for signs and listen to the baby's heart rate, and (3) the healthiness of our house for birthing. These concerns were answered by Charity's studies. I even studied the materials she brought home. These included emergency birthing guides, *William's Obstetrics,* and other stuff.

While Charity is laboring, I usually feel like a heel. I am tired, but not as tired as she is. I am uncomfortable; she, more. I want to take a nap; she is too uncomfortable to. I watch her pain and rub her back and wish that I had not made her have to hurt like this. I feel this even though I know that she won't care about the pain in a few hours. I try to distract myself with little tasks.

When really heavy labor is going on, I experience a few more intense emotions. I remember one birth where the contractions were so intense that Charity began to shudder with some of them. I got choked up; she was tough. It was kind of like watching a John Wayne movie for the first time. I think, "I love you." I can't do anything more than I am, keeping pressure on her back and praying; maybe a little hug now and again.

We keep checking the baby's heart rate, and Charity's blood pressure and heart rate. As long as they don't show too great a fluctuation, I don't get scared. When the baby is moving through the birth canal, there is not really time to worry too much. The contractions are so rapid and I am just trying to keep Charity happy and help her breathe.

During the births of our children, my major apprehensions center around Charity. I want to be able to get her to help, or vice versa, if she needs it. It usually isn't until after the baby crowns that I am concerned for the baby.

The second and fourth births had a really short time between crowning and the head being born. When she is crowning, I am saying, "Don't push, don't push, breathe, breathe." I am concerned that it go slowly enough that she not tear or rupture. She is saying, "I'm not pushing; my body is." Those two babies came so fast from crowning to the birth of the head that I did not have time to worry—here is this slippery little baby squirting out at me.

When the head has been born, I check for the cord around the baby's neck and tell Charity that it is not there (this has been her concern). Then I encourage her to wait a contraction or so and then push.

When our new gift is in my hands, I check for sex, then breathing. The sex of the baby isn't really important, but for some reason, that's what gets looked into first. After I know that the baby is breathing, I am okay. I check for fingers and toes, color, spine, and the roof of the mouth.

I give Charity the baby and start with the cord stuff, and then the placenta. She wants to push. I say let your body and the placenta do it itself. She either gives the baby her breast or applies nipple stimulation to encourage contractions. After all this, I check the placenta for completeness. "Now, how are we bleeding? Massage that thing. Harder."

After everybody has held the new gift, I hold him / her a little. After thanking God and getting choked up, I clean up. And when that's done, everybody leaves, and we take a very happy nap: mom, dad and baby.

Peter

Judie woke me up early on the morning of April 29th. I was sound asleep, so when she woke me up I was quite groggy. When I heard her say it was time, everything in my body went onto an alert state. I quickly dressed (and made sure I put my sneakers on so I wouldn't slip on any fluids…. I know, what was I thinking?) I ran into the bathroom just in time to see Judie's water break on the floor.

I think it was about at this point that I felt like someone else was taking control of my hands. Things started to happen so quickly that I didn't have time to really think or analyze, which was actually better for me in my frame of mind. As I walked Judie back into our bedroom, I remember thinking, "I have to get my sterilized surgeon's gloves on," but when I tried to put on a couple of different pairs, I just ripped them to shreds. Judie placed her hands on our computer desk and began to bear down. I got underneath and witnessed what appeared to be a very strange sight at first. The butt end of my son, Dylan popped out, and one leg dropped down. I remained quiet and did not tell Judie about the positioning of our first son. A couple moments passed and his second leg, which was folded up against his chest, still had not come down. I reached over to help it down, but just as I was about to touch it, it came out on its own. I was amazed.

Then I watched his torso slide out and arm flop down. His left arm seemed to be stuck. Once again, I thought he needed assistance. I gently pulled down, and his arm, with the pressure on it, seemed to snap down and slap his leg. I thought I might have actually broken it, but thank God there was no problem at all. The rest of him (up to his forehead) slid out rather easily. At this point, I thought I might have to help again. I tried to massage Judie's perineum, but she said not to. After another moment or two, Dylan came all the way out.

Man, was this fantastic!...to actually hold him and witness his first breath. It was about ten seconds later, that Dylan's placenta forcefully splashed down onto the floor, but Dylan was safe in my arms. Here is where Judie and my accounts differ a little. I remember asking Judie to step back as I held Dylan in my right arm. Judie stepped back close to our bed and began to deliver the second baby, Luke. I looked down and saw a large, clear-white substance, which looked like a giant egg-white. It wasn't breaking, so I gingerly pulled it away from her vagina. Luke immediately came out after. He was also butt first and there were no delays. I caught him in my left arm and set Dylan down on the bed, wrapped in a towel. I was then able to hold Luke with both hands. Luke's umbilical cord and placenta were still inside Judie and they did not come out as quickly. Judie finally sat down, and after a couple of minutes, she was able to expel in a bucket.

I wiped off the babies and began to feel my system slow down a little. Jared, my oldest son came in the room at this point and made sure that Luke wasn't going to fall off the bed. After about 25-30 minutes, I tied the babies' cords and cut them with a pair of sterilized scissors.

I remember thinking a couple of days later, how during this whole experience, I seemed to "zone out" mentally. I just remember doing all the right things, almost as if Jesus took over my hands and mind, so I wouldn't do anything stupid. I also recall, reading out loud, Bible verses which we had posted around the walls of our room. This seemed to help a great deal. The next two weeks I took off were relaxing mentally, if not physically. I was doing a lot of housework, but I wasn't thinking anything about my job, nor did I have the burden of concern about the births any longer.

As I reflect now, it almost seems like a dream I had. How anything with such potential for something to go wrong could turn out so smoothly and so easily, just *has* to be a miracle of Jesus Christ. I really give Him credit. He really has become more and more the Peace of my family. It truly is a wonderful thing to have such a powerful experience of Christ's faithfulness to reflect back and even anchor onto at times. It is also quite inspiring for His future care, no matter what. I know Jesus Christ is always with us in a real, spiritual way.

When third parties muscle in between husband and wife, a disruption occurs in the marriage relationship with tragic consequences. The birthing mom's attention is diverted from her husband to the midwife with the result that mom becomes bonded to her. For decades women have been falling in love with their doctors. Now, they're falling in love with their midwives, with dad again being left out in the cold. —Marilyn Moran

10

Self-Actualization

We are all functioning at a small fraction of our capacity to live fully in its total meaning of loving, caring, creating and adventuring. Consequently, the actualizing of our potential can become the most exciting adventure of our lifetime.
—Herbert Otto

Life, liberty and the pursuit of happiness. Happiness means different things to different people, but whether or not our basic needs are met, we all want to be happy. Though many people seek success in their work and personal lives, they may not be truly fulfilled until their goals are achieved and a sense of accomplishment has been realized. Others seek to please themselves physically, materially or socially, satisfying themselves with passing time immersed in activities and not feeling a need to set and pursue goals.

Rite of passage

During our lifetime, we will experience several milestones or rites of passage. These events are opportunities for tremendous growth and serve as a transition to another stage of life. High school graduation, moving away from home, college graduation, a new job or career, marriage, and birth of a child bring mixed emotions of exhilaration, apprehension and anxiety. When confidence in our abilities is put to the test, we will undoubtedly emerge a new person.

The birth of a child is perhaps the most significant event in a couple's life. The experience of childbirth can contribute to the initial attachment of the parents to the newborn and intensify the couple's feelings toward each other. Birth for single parents or in the absence of one's spouse is just as much a rite of passage for an individual as it is for the married couple.

Rites of passage include three phases: *separation, transition and return.* Separation from society or others prepares us for the beginning of a personal transformation. Sometimes we may feel lonely, as if we are the only one in the world experiencing the milestone. This feeling leads us to become apprehensive, excited and anxious all at once as we prepare for high school graduation, our wedding day or child's birth. The rite of passage requires an initial separation in order to prepare for changes to come. If you discuss your plans to have an unassisted homebirth with people who have opposing viewpoints, you may have a hard time detaching yourself as you prepare for the transition.

This transition involves tasks which will be faced successfully or unsuccessfully. If we feel successful after going through a rite of passage, we will complete an event with confidence and be mentally returned to life feeling like a "new" person, but if the rite of passage was unsuccessful, we may not feel a sense of balance or completion.

Peak experience

> In states of peak experience, we experience phenomena in their simplicity, 'oughtness,' beauty, goodness, and completeness. There is a lack of strain, an effortlessness, a spontaneity about the experience that is almost overwhelming. Typically there is a lack of space and time. Intense emotions such as wonder, awe, and reverence are felt. During

The tragedy of love is indifference. —Somerset Maugham

these intense experiences, individuals transcend their own selfishness. Events and objects are perceived as they truly are and are not distorted to meet the experiencers' needs or wishes.   (Ryckman 1982: 371)

When you read the birth stories presented in this book or talk to those who have had DIY births, you will notice that several men and women lost track of time during the birth. Childbirth is experienced as a simple, natural event and it takes less effort than couples are led to believe.

What takes effort, straining and struggling at other times is now done without any sense of striving, of working or laboring, but 'comes of itself.' One sees the appearance of calm sureness and rightness, as if they knew exactly what they were doing, and were doing it wholeheartedly, without doubts, equivocations, hesitations or partial withdrawal. (Maslow 1968: 106)

The person in peak-experiences feels himself, more than at other times, to be the responsible, active, creating center of his activities and of his perceptions. He feels more like a prime mover, more self-determined (rather than caused, determined, helpless, dependent, passive, weak, bossed). He feels himself to be his own boss, fully responsible, fully volitional, with more 'free will' than at other times, master of his fate, an agent.   (Maslow 1968: 107)

It is difficult, if not impossible to reach a peak birth experience in a hospital. Most women are not aware of the possibility of a birth orgasm or that birth can be pleasant. Women need to organize themselves mentally while orienting themselves externally, to physical surroundings. It is necessary to push aside anything that is irrelevant to having the baby. Try doing it in a hospital, where you are distracted by people, demands, smells, room temperature and discomforts. It is almost impossible to reach a necessary level of detachment, making birth, under those circumstances, an inhibition and exhibition rather than an adventure.

Self-Actualization

Unassisted homebirthers often achieve what psychologist Abraham Maslow described as self-actualization. Many couples recognize themselves in the following description:

> The self-actualizing individual, by definition gratified in his basic needs, is far less dependent, far less beholden, far more autonomous and self-directed. Far from needing other people, growth-motivated people may actually be hampered by them.... The determinants which govern them are now primarily inner ones, rather than social or environmental. They are the laws of their own inner nature, their potentialities and capacities, their talents, their latent resources, their creative impulses, their needs to know themselves and to become more and more integrated and unified, more and more aware of what they really are, of what they really want, of what their call or vocation or fate is to be. (Maslow 1968: 34)

Although most of the men whose stories appear in this book read something about the anatomy and physiology of birth, cord clamping and responding to minor problems, their instincts during the birth dominated intellectual preparation. When instincts served as their guide, they did not perceive a cord wrapped around the baby's neck as an emergency. Instead, they simply lifted it over the baby's head and helped their wives complete their mission. There was no panic, no sense of effort, but a sense of tranquillity at their births.

Traditional childbirth does not lend itself to self-actualization. "If the environment is restrictive and minimizes personal choice, the individual is likely to develop in neurotic ways since this inner nature is weak and subject to control by environmental forces." (Ryckman 1982: 365) The hospital environment imposes its rules upon nature. The cultural environment is restrictive when a majority of couples do not even consider an option other than prenatal care with an OB/Gyn, culminating in a hospital delivery.

How birth experiences can leave us psychologically incomplete

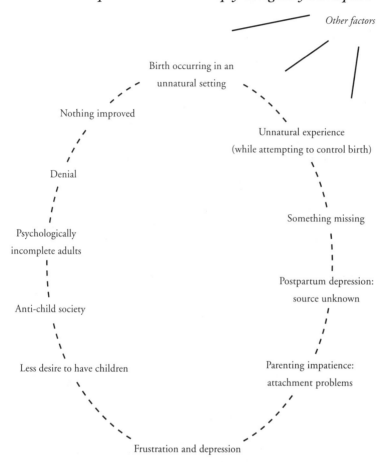

A lot of research has been done regarding anxiety and depression, postpartum depression and mental health. Because it is a major event which alters life, childbearing has an impact on mental health. Birth experiences affect psychological "completeness" in adulthood. Postpartum adjustment, confidence and ease in parental roles, and the desire for more children are affected by a couple's birth experience. Ideas presented here are the result of conversations with and observations of hundreds of parents.

The progression of stages does not occur without interference. Environmental factors may enter at any time. For example, a poor birth experience is not the only cause of frustration and depression. A couple may have had several unnatural birth experiences, but it does not mean that they will develop anti-child attitudes. Outcomes are a result of experiences and interpretations of events. Environmental factors may contribute to internal changes. New ideas and coping strategies can enable people to depart this paradigm at any time and at any stage.

It is very difficult for a birth to unfold naturally and comfortably when it takes place in an unnatural setting. Some couples may never fully adjust to the hospital environment. Medical attendants are free to do whatever is necessary to ensure the delivery of a child. As often as women submit themselves to this ritual and force themselves to accept it, it is still a very uncomfortable experience. Whether the woman is uninhibited or shy is irrelevant. Birth brings out the sense of modesty and privacy in most people.

An unnatural experience occurs when a woman gives birth in a physically uncomfortable position or uses drugs to control the labor. The baby is welcomed into an artificial environment. Couples may not recognize their experience as unnatural unless they have another birth which they can compare.

Some new mothers may not feel as if anything was missing from their birth experience because it is difficult to pinpoint what was lacking from a birth experience which resulted in a healthy newborn. Some doctors and hospital staffs manage births as something to endure, depriving women of the opportunity to enjoy their births.

It is not surprising that postpartum depression is common among new mothers. Many women continue the same level of household chores and family responsibilities even though sleep patterns are interrupted. People do not question whether the birth caused postpartum blues, but believe that their depression can be attributed to a "difficult" baby. When the baby will not sleep, nurse, or quiet down, it is the baby's behavior they seek to change, when what needs readjustment are the mothers' attitudes. The newborn is a disruption to former daily routines, and the mother often lacks adequate support that could benefit her in the early days and beyond.

Attachment and bonding problems accompany postpartum depression, because separations between mother and newborn are regular events in the hospital. Immediately following birth, the baby is taken away to be cleaned, measured and observed. The breastfeeding experience may be challenging if the nursery staff keeps the baby in their care, causing touching and caressing of the new baby to be less frequent in the hospital environment. Mothers who are going through a period of depression are usually focused on their needs and may be impatient caring for their newborn.

Although it may take several weeks or months for the stress or depression to subside, as the depression does lift, the parents begin to enjoy their baby more. They are sometimes not as willing to have another child if they remember the first few months of their previous baby's life as burdensome. Given the circumstances, who would want to go through another pregnancy and hospital birth? Many couples wait several years before getting the courage to enter the world of assembly-line obstetrics and hospital delivery a second time.

Couples internalize negative ideas about children from a society comprised of self-centered people, especially since some aggressively dissuade large families. Children are seen as planned choices that interfere with rather than enhance life. Most people believe that having children is not only an economic consideration, but a major investment in time and energy, and from this selfish perspective, children are burdens rather than gifts. Because many people are not able to fully embrace the total joy that children bring to their lives, obstetricians are eager to prescribe birth control or perform

> A healthy soul shines through the persona on most days and blazes through on others. —Clarissa Pinkola Estes

surgeries to block conception after a couple has three or four children. It is as if pregnancy and childbirth is special for a first-time mother or for someone whose second child is of a different sex.

Couples with several children are likely to hear negative, insensitive comments such as, "Wow, your hands are full!...How do you do it?...Better you than me....Are you going to have any more kids?...Are all of those kids yours?...Haven't you figured out how to prevent that from happening?...There are things you can do to stop having kids, you know...." It is not as common, but refreshing to hear remarks like, "Wow! What a nice family....Your children are so beautiful and well behaved." Parents with several adult children seldom regretted having raised large families, because there is such a sense of accomplishment after having struggled.

Families are smaller today and children are segregated from the adult world. There is an emphasis on engaging in activities within the same age group. Parents want to provide their children with as many experiences as possible. Many parents know that they will only be able to do a good job with no more than two children. It is hard to balance work, family and personal aspirations with several children.

Part of a happy, healthy adulthood involves the ability not to take life so seriously, to laugh a lot and to enjoy the kind of spontaneity that children do. Adults who participate in child's play have an easier time of expressing their inner child, especially those who have a large family and are involved with their children's lives and cannot escape spontaneous play with their children. Adults who are childless or lack a sense of spontaneity are missing a part of life which contributes to creativity and well-being. Having a large family or embracing children keeps adults young. Unfortunately, there is a segment of our population that is unable to derive any pleasure or fun because they are much too serious and psychologically incomplete.

Life can be very pressuring for parents raising children. Not only does everyone want the best education for their children, but they want them to grow up healthy in a safe, peaceful world. We have certain expectations and worries about the future, causing us to set limits or visualize a certain family size.

People who have a pessimistic view of life may not aim for a satisfying birth, especially when the main goal of childbirth is a healthy outcome, and all else is secondary. Women adopt low standards or no standards for a satisfying birth experience. When birth experiences do not go so well for the mother, they are discounted, as if a healthy newborn justifies ignoring a pitiful birth experience. And if the newborn is not so healthy, friends and family discuss the current problems and how things could be worse, totally ignoring the birth experience.

Remaining trapped in denial means that improvements will not occur, and the couple will return to the hospital for a repeat performance in a few years. Conversely, couples who have had unassisted homebirths have often achieved a level of self-actualization they know can never be attained in a hospital environment, making it highly unlikely that they will ever return to that sterile environment where the beauty of birth is more likely to be taken away than freely and joyfully experienced.

Unassisted homebirth: a lonely choice

Society imposes many restrictions upon us, making it difficult to experience life on our own terms if we are bombarded by employers, friends, significant others, family and strangers telling us what we should do and how we must live. "Society" is a collection of individuals with different values, interests, and talents. A handful of individuals, not "society," is partially restraining us from doing what we would like to do and being who we would like to be. It is more manageable to fend off distracting influences in our lives when we can pinpoint the source. *We* decide what we want to think or how we want to react towards others. *We* are ultimately restraining ourselves from attaining our dreams.

Being *fully alive* and involved with life means being open to new experiences and sometimes committed to unpopular beliefs, striving for new directions and new awakenings, breaking old patterns, creating a vivid sense of self. At the same time, we search for order and harmony in the universe. Self-inquiry may shake up the foundation and threaten the harmony we are searching for. Self-inquiry is a painful process, and what was formerly accepted is suddenly questioned. Even though man seeks consistency, he still strives for perfection, knowledge, truth and awareness. But uncertainty, insecurity, restlessness and new awakenings are the ultimate realities of human existence.

The denial of our deepest self is a denial of life. We are not living life to its fullest when we do not strive for expression of our inner needs. We should not have to sacrifice what our inner voice is telling us. We can make many choices in life about the way we want to be. Ultimately, no one or nothing can destroy our inner peace, for the greater the inner peace, the more peaceful our outer world. If we live with love and high standards in our hearts and minds, no one can get us to change our integrity—to lie, cheat, steal, or degrade another person. When we have attained a comfortable level of inner peace, we may feel separate from others, but it will not bother us.

Birth pioneers are those who make lonely, unpopular choices as they seek beauty, grace and fulfillment in the life-giving process. They strive for improvements for themselves and future generations. Unassisted homebirth lends itself perfectly to self-actualization and is the springboard for a deeper, richer life.

To be ourselves causes us to be exiled by many others, and yet to comply with what others want causes us to be exiled from ourselves. —Clarissa Pinkola Estes

PART III

Pain and Suffering

11

The Many Forces
Against Us

Average or neurotic people will fear much that lies within
themselves. They control, they inhibit, they repress, and
they suppress. They disapprove of their deeper selves and
expect that others do, too. (Maslow 1968: 141)

Many people are uneasy with the idea of unassisted homebirth and still others would prefer that any thought or mention of unassisted birth be eliminated. The main reasons
involve misconceptions of childbirth, economic threat, ego
and power threats. Discomfort and denial of childbirth alternatives are based on FEAR, "False Expectations About
Reality." It is in the best interests of those with power to
persuade the less powerful that homebirth is unsafe and inferior.

Those who oppose

(1) Medical professionals

In addition to obstetricians and midwives, opposition
comes from neonatologists, anesthesiologists, obstetrical
nurses and pediatricians. It is easy to see that medical specialists who routinely witness women who are unhealthy,

afraid, or want to eliminate pain, will, themselves come to see birth as painful and risky. Even if the evidence supports that birth will be normal and problem-free in most cases, they have a hard time believing it. Normalcy has become so redefined that they oppose anything outside their norm.

(2) Insurance companies

Insurance companies are in business to make money. Since maternity payouts do not exceed the premiums that are collected, the companies do not lose money and there is little incentive to reevaluate a system that is successful. Since insurance companies profit, they convince the public that they too are profiting from excellent maternity coverage.

Executives, managers and employees of insurance companies are members of a society that firmly agrees with the childbirth myths (see Chapter 6). Insurance companies consist of individuals who assume that women and babies are safest in hospitals with a highly paid medical staff and superior technology, and their customer base agrees.

> Facts have little power to sway opinion....No one is truly neutral, and decisions are made on emotion and tradition, not on logic and facts....We seem to have a very illogical situation of countless women submitting their bodies and their newborn babies to a system which consistently fails to provide them comfort, safety or service for which they pay for so dearly. (Balizet 1996: 140)

Insurance companies could save millions of dollars if coverage included midwife-attended homebirth. While it appears that more money would be saved if couples chose unassisted homebirth, the insurance companies might actually lose money. Couples who are self-reliant might not even opt to pay premiums for benefits they will not use.

(3) Childbirth educators

Perhaps self-employed childbirth educators would be supportive of men and women choosing unassisted birth. After all, childbirth educators are not bound by organizations which impose an economic or philosophical bias. The only opposition would be a personal one which would reveal their agreement with the myths of childbirth or an unwillingness to take a stand for unpopular choices. Even the most progressive Bradley instructors refused to attend or help a friend of mine at her unassisted birth. They claimed that their reputations were at stake, but I believe that they fear unassisted homebirth.

After my unassisted birth, a childbirth educator and midwife asked me the same question that others often ask: "So, everything went all right?" This question implies that something will go wrong with birth. It is a question asked when someone is pessimistic, has low expectations, or a lack of faith. Their implications and generalizations were based on experiences with problematic births. They are searching for one couple whose answer is, "No, everything did not turn out okay." They are looking for one response that will validate their assumption that unassisted homebirth is not safe or desirable.

(4) Society at large

Many married women are occupied with careers, lead busy lives, or do not spend much time in the home. Their source of information on pregnancy, childbirth and childrearing comes from medical professionals. Since past generations are not communicating quality childbirth information to the next generations, doctors and other paid experts are sought. Although there is a lot of information about childbirth alternatives, women are not likely to spend any time looking for it and fall prey to the obstetrics and gynecology bias. The American College of Obstetrics and Gynecology does not recommend ultrasound for routine pregnancies, yet very few offices follow that guideline. There are people who practice non-traditional medicine, but they are harder to find and smaller in number. Women who seek alternatives are questioned by their friends and families. People who claim to be open-minded wonder why a couple would have an unassisted homebirth when this country has the best technology and experts to deliver babies.

If economics is not a factor, why are people opposed to unassisted homebirth? Do they really care? Are they concerned about safety? Or are they threatened by someone's ability to be uninhibited? Are they envious or perhaps doubtful of their own ability to give birth? If they are fearful, they may feel that others should be fearful too.

We all know people who are unhappy and who cannot be joyous for others. Depressed and withdrawn, some people are too preoccupied with their own problems to notice what's going on around them. People who have competitive thoughts and behaviors may try to diminish others' happiness or goals.

Many women suffer from a poor body image, shame or guilt, and may not feel worthy or deserving of an intimate birth. Men and women make birth choices based on their upbringing and social expectations, some seeking to deny others the opportunity to make choices.

Our beloved family and friends

Some people depend on the encouragement and approval of family and friends. Often, family members who are aware of the couple's plan for an unassisted homebirth are the biggest opponents. Not only do they fear for the couple, but they may even develop anger and hostility toward the couple.

Of course, it is wonderful when family and friends share in the excitement and anticipation. The extended family may be invited to witness one of life's most beautiful events. One young couple who was living with a couple in their mid-fifties revealed their plans to have an unassisted homebirth. It seemed as if everyone supported their plans, but when labor started, the young couple felt pressured to go to the hospital. Orders and threats turned to reality when someone called police and emergency medical service to the scene. The birth couple simply got in their car and traveled to a friend's house to complete the birth. The friend had previously given birth without assistance and understood what was necessary for a peaceful birth.

Our sexually dysfunctional society

Our country has an abundance of noncommittal sexual relationships as well as an increasing number of sexually related crimes. Cohabitation, casual sex and one night stands are the epitome of sexual selfishness, which does not usually contribute to a stable society. Outcomes include prostitution, extramarital sex, abortion, sexually transmitted diseases, acceptance of pornography, incest, and other obsessions and deviancies.

When you look at how civilized our country is and then you look at all of the problems related to sex, you have to wonder just how civilized we really are. Many people are complacent about teenage pregnancy, out of wedlock babies, abortion, surrogate parenting, fertility drugs, in vitro fertilization, pornography, prostitution, adultery, and sexually transmitted diseases. Cohabitation, homosexuality, crossdressing and unions between partners of an age difference wide enough to be a parent-child situation are not seen as deviant behavior, but alternative choices. Those who are not tolerant and accepting of the whole spectrum of life styles are accused of narrow-mindedness and insensitivity. Standards for sexual behavior become so low that there seems to be no baseline for mature, acceptable behavior.

The desire to control exactly how many children we will have and when we will have them is a way of life. Anxiety and disappointment occur when things do not go our way. Those who have had problems conceiving a child see nothing wrong or unusual with manipulating science for their benefit. Fertility drugs, artificial insemination, in vitro fertilization and surrogate parenting are not considered abnormal by many. They are simply possibilities that science offers.

I know a couple who achieved a multiple pregnancy after taking fertility drugs. The doctor recommended that one fetus be aborted so that the other two would have a better chance of survival. After careful consideration, the couple had the procedure done. Most people who know them are grateful for what science has done; they are the proud parents of twins.

The images in our culture portray sex as fun and pleasurable, which it is. However, without an equal emphasis on consequences and responsibility, the results can be disastrous. Focusing on physical pleasure and disregarding any goal outside of physical sensation allows for anything and everything. Not only are there unwanted children and inconvenient diseases to contend with, but there are also problems in relationships. An overemphasis on glamorous sex often leaves women feeling physically inferior; they are unable to compete with the images of perfection depicted on television, in movies and in magazines.

Dissatisfaction with appearance or sexuality contributes to insecurity in giving birth. Emphasis on being thin or shapely does not help an insecure woman feel confident and beautiful during pregnancy and birth. It does not matter what the rest of the world thinks about a woman's pregnancy. It's only crucial that a woman feel good enough about her body in the presence of her mate. Yes, there may be times where women might want to lose a few pounds or get in shape, but if they are distraught about their body, they may not want to open themselves up (pun intended) for an intimate birth experience.

You would think that a society which enjoys sexual freedoms should have many sexually uninhibited individuals. Too many people are not willing to let go of the need for order and control. The sterile way women give birth in this country and the low incidence of breastfeeding are indicative of inhibitions about sexuality. It is unfortunate that many women do not surrender during birth, the pinnacle of their sexuality.

Other unassisted homebirthers

Since unassisted homebirth is not a common practice, you would think that those who have shared this experience would feel an affinity toward each other. That is not necessarily true. As with anything in life, people can be opinionated, intolerant or feel that one way is superior to others. Often the lines are drawn in the religious arena. Christians who believe that there is only one true way of living life have a hard time embracing a Buddhist couple who describe the spiritual, emotional and physical benefits of an unassisted homebirth. "New Age" homebirthers might dismiss homebirthers with strong Christian beliefs even if an exchange of ideas could benefit everyone concerned. Couples may have been very moved by the experience; they may be very happy and fulfilled in their marriage, family life and religious practices, yet a common bond may not even exist.

Emotions run strong among people who feel that their ideas for a perfect birth are superior to others. Many believe that a husband and wife birth is the desired goal. Some may disapprove of an unmarried woman birthing her baby with her ten year-old daughter, while others may feel birth is primarily about a woman striving for complete autonomy. Still, others may adhere to dogmas and disagree with the view that a successful birth is best defined by each particular woman or couple.

If spiritual philosophies divide unassisted homebirthers, psychological considerations often unite them. Many women want to birth a baby in a loving manner, with total self-acceptance, free from inhibitions. DIYers believe that pregnancy and birth are safe, while the general public assumes pregnancy and birth are unsafe.

Life entails many complexities and one way we give meaning to our world is by generalizing. It is easier for us to categorize. Classifying people into groups requires little or no explanation. An understanding of individuality is sacrificed when people simplify. People are described as Republican or Democrat, Christian or non-Christian, American or foreigner, black or white. Just as there exists a whole spectrum of variation, the same holds true for those who have unassisted homebirths. Conflict and disagreement occur within any group.

It is not necessary for unassisted homebirthers to form a common bond, but it is important that we allow room for various ideas about birthing. We should all rejoice when we hear of a couple who discovers unassisted birth, for it usually brings great joy and personal growth to everyone involved.

"How can you be so irresponsible?"

"Why would you want to have a baby at home?" and "How can you be so irresponsible?" Those are questions asked by people who believe the myths of childbirth. Couples who choose to have an unassisted homebirth make a bold, courageous decision that requires effort—effort to assure a healthy pregnancy and a safe birth and effort to persevere amidst negative cultural forces. Couples must be focused, reasonably sure of their decision, knowledgeable about the physiology of birth and newborns, and consider contingency plans. Obviously, unassisted birth requires goal-setting and foresight. It is not a rebellious act against establishment, but rather a quest for a satisfying birth.

When you choose a doctor, he will diagnose and treat problems. He is responsible for the birth. The mother who chooses an unassisted homebirth seeks to eliminate and prevent problems in the first place. That is being responsible.

Some homebirthers may be dismissed as eccentric and lacking common sense. Those who pursue unassisted birth have usually spent much time contemplating the hows and whys of their decision.

Crime and punishment

Those who do not conform to the system are sometimes given a hard time by those entrenched in the system or those with power. Take for example the birth certificate. When a woman gives birth in a hospital, the standard procedure is for the paperwork to be done the next day. The doctor takes credit for the delivery and that is the end of that. A woman who has not had prenatal care and delivered the baby at home may have to go to extreme measures to get a birth certificate. She must prove the baby is actually hers.

Bureaucracies are cognitively challenged when an unusual case comes across their desk. A friend of mine had to hire a lawyer because she did not apply for the birth certificate within five days of her baby's birth. Another woman had a hard time because her letters verifying pregnancy from her chiropractor and a Birthright facility were unacceptable. In order to obtain a birth certificate, she was told she needed a letter signed by an M.D.

My doctor refused to release my medical records or sign a statement verifying my pregnancy unless I paid him $50.00. I felt that this was unreasonable, so I asked my primary care physician for my records which verified the pregnancy. I also had some resistance from her office, but eventually got her cooperation. It's as if I broke a taboo and had to be punished for it.

After a while, I felt like withdrawing from life and my emotional reaction was, "It's negative to have children and why am I going through all of this?" Then I would stop feeling sorry for myself and feel comforted knowing that life entails many struggles. I knew I was not going to be let down in the end and would emerge a stronger person.

Local doctors and midwives did not care to give a friend of mine a postpartum appointment because she had an unassisted homebirth. She was in need of medical attention and was finally able to schedule an appointment two weeks later. Another woman developed an infection due to a retained amniotic sac.

I was refused medical treatment at a Medchoice center and the only hospital in town that has an obstetric ward. I could have gone to the emergency room at another hospital, but I feared sitting in the waiting room all night, hostile treatment, being sent to the hospital that had already refused me, having a flunky doctor wanting to do a D&C or hysterectomy. My CNM saw me first thing the next day and treated the problem with a simple vaginal exam and antibiotics. She is located seventy miles away in another town. My family doctor later told me he would have treated me too. Both were disgusted with how I was treated. Interestingly, both went against their peers in providing me with prenatal care. I guess for every 100 bad ones, there are at least two saints.

I have had no success grabbing the attention of psychologists or marriage counselors with my insights about the role of birth in bonding husband and wife. Dr. Ratner did say once that he is on my wavelength. Other than that, everyone has turned a deaf ear to what I'm saying. I guess Thomas Kuhn is correct—that specialists are so fixated on the present thinking, they have no desire to explore anything new. It just takes time for others (like the laity) to investigate alternate possibilities and eventually the 'specialists' quietly climb aboard, or else they just die off and there is no one left but those who have explored the new evidence and accepted it, rejecting the former way which had been so entrenched. —Marilyn Moran

12

Who Needs Doctors?

> The fact that you're there in the first place means you don't
> know *how* you are or what is going on with *you* and that
> you want the doctor to tell you. So you're ready to give up
> a precious liberty, that of self-identification....The doctor
> sets the limits of what's normal and abnormal, what's good
> and what's bad. (Mendelsohn 1982: 36)

Dr. Michael Benson, author of *Birth Day!* states that OB/
Gyn's are needed for 3 reasons: (1) for reassurance and emotional support (2) to relieve pain and (3) to intervene in the
rare cases where the mother's or baby's life is at risk. Reading this book made me realize that I did not need a doctor
during childbirth, because *Birth Day!* approached birth me-
chanically and seemed incomplete, the tone was patronizing
and the beauty of birth was totally missing from its pages.

My expertise extends to me and my family; I do not pro-
claim to be an expert in the area of childbirth, nor do I wish
to serve as an obstetrician or midwife at other births. Unassisted homebirthers do not seek to replace the field of obstetrics, but humbly choose a different manner of birthing.
Obstetrics is an important specialty that has a place in the
medical field.

Many Americans do not hire a chef to cook their meals,
or employ a personal trainer to manage their exercise program, or hire an accountant to do their taxes. Women seek

doctors to deliver their babies because they perceive child-birth to be something complex rather than something that is a simple process.

When we view childbirth as a straightforward process in which couples can gain skills to bear their own children in a natural setting, we realize that birth is not as complex as we are led to believe. Each one of us has the opportunity to become self-sufficient in almost any area of life.

In sickness and in health

When do you go to a doctor? Only when you are ill? Many people go to the doctor's office when they are well. Semi-annual dental appointments, annual visits to the gyne-cologist or optometrist, well baby checks, annual physicals and follow-up appointments infringe upon our time. They undermine confidence and responsibility for ourselves.

Some seek doctors for help or to appease a family member. Others use doctors to alleviate fears and insecurities.

Seeking a doctor to help cure an illness or alleviate a problem should be the last effort after exhausting other resources and options, but many people turn to doctors at the mere hint of any problem before searching for their own answers. Year after year obstetricians handle predominantly healthy, routine pregnancies and deliveries, and yet they are surgeon-specialists. There is no medical reason why more couples could not deliver their own children at home.

Doctors thrive when their expertise is fully challenged by a patient's problem. They can then feel the most useful as they draw on all of their experience to treat a problem suc-cessfully. I am sure that none of my four different obstetri-cians would remember me, my pregnancies or deliveries be-cause they were "uneventful." In fact, they probably could not even picture me and would have difficulty remembering me if they were to review their precious charts.

Excellent health should be a goal for everyone. Few people desire poor health. While peace of mind and physical com-fort can be gained through consultations with doctors, patients need to understand that there are instances where doctors are only able to offer "trial and error" solutions.

Opposing goals

> Most of a woman's depressions, ennuis, and wandering confusions are caused by a severely restricted soul-life in which innovation, impulse, and creation are restricted or forbidden. Women receive enormous impulse to act from the creative force. We cannot overlook the fact that there is still much thieving and hamstringing of women's talents through cultural restriction and punishment of her natural wildish instincts. (Estes 1992: 274)

Many doctors assume that women are not medically interested or knowledgeable and that one goal of childbirth is to escape physical pain. It is true that many women want their doctors to make decisions for them, but the overuse of technology, adherence to medical dogmas, and reliance on tests detract from the specialness of pregnancy and birth. Women are not encouraged to take responsibility for themselves because if they did, they would not need the establishment. Submission to authority is expected and the authority often abuses its power, both intentionally and unintentionally.

1. Optimist meets pessimist

The first thing a healthy pregnant woman does is seek a doctor's care. She arrives upbeat and enthusiastic to her first office visit. The doctor is looking for a problem to diagnose, almost hoping to find a malady. The medical system supports the doctor's philosophy.

> ...medical institutions, medical drug manufacturers, medical device industries, and medical professionals, in general, receive their benefits and their incomes in an amount proportional to the abundance of abnormality, sickness and complications. (Stewart 1997: 23)

Over the course of several months, the doctor's apathy and pessimism replaces some of the patient's optimism to the extent that she is monitoring herself for problems. Unbeknownst to this patient, the doctor's and hospital's goals of birth will be adopted by her. A woman who enters the birth institution thinking she will have a completely natural experience had better be an intensely persistent woman.

2. Protector versus encourager

Man feels a strong need to protect a woman during vulnerable moments. What better time than pregnancy and birth is there for a man to assist the woman? Rather than a doctor or midwife assisting, the woman should look no farther than her husband. Problems arise when the protector does not fully understand the needs of who he is protecting. While the birthing mother needs to be protected from physical and emotional interference, the protector's (doctor's) perceptions and external constraints of his profession contribute to his choice of solutions and treatments of what he believes to be the problem, never really understanding the birthing mothers true needs.

While acting solely as a protector, a doctor misses the opportunity to act as an encourager, whereas a lover deeply knows who he is protecting and, because he is not distracted by external rules, he can also encourage his partner. There is no question that his motives are pure. An added benefit of encouragement is that it can lead to ecstasy.

> So the modern obstetrician's attitude toward birth is cautious to the extreme. When he looks at birth he is waiting for something to go wrong. Pain is the assumption from which he works, for the obstetrician not only believes in the truth of pain in labor, he subconsciously or consciously suggests this pain to the woman he assists. His image of woman is that of a fragile, emotional creature not meant to endure strenuous work or pain. He likens her to a child, and through excessive and misplaced sympathy, he seeks

to spare this grown-up little girl any suffering in the course
of birth. (Arms 1975: 120)

3. Want versus need

Women *want* to have a baby and medical professionals
need to make themselves useful. Even though most doctors
want to help their patients, pregnant women who desire a
natural birth should try to estimate their doctor's level of respect for nature, attempting to assess, for example, how long
the doctor will wait before intervening. The woman's wants
and the doctor's needs may be at odds.

Doctors rely on technology and tests to make determinations. Technology in their minds is a means to an end, so it
is a problem when there are no patients who need the high
tech equipment or worse, when patients are considered a
means to make money.

> That many women feel they have failed in one way or an-
> other in their births is not due to the method they practice
> but to the expectation of failure built into every hospital
> staff. It is this patronizing, negative attitude—more than
> the technology that spawns it—that makes natural child-
> birth a deception in the modern hospital. If women were
> to succeed at having their babies spontaneously and in un-
> complicated fashion, requiring only assistance and not in-
> tervention, then the hospital staff, trained in crisis and dis-
> ease, would find itself with nothing medically to do. (Arms
> 1975: 142)

4. Matter over mind

Did you ever notice that when you go to your obstetrician, you will not hear the empowering words, "Let's do everything we can to have a satisfying birth experience"? He

> A doctor anesthetizes himself through anesthetizing a
> woman, in order to avoid his own fears about pain. - Helen
> Watkins

knows how to deal with you as a patient with a condition, an illness, and not as a woman with deep emotions as you go through pregnancy, one of the most joyous times in your life. The mom in anticipation is feeling the wonder, awe and miracle of life, but even the most enthusiastic and dedicated doctor has a hard time sharing this joy with one of his patients.

OB/Gyns focus on the physical elements of birth and exclude the psychological and emotional aspects, which impact couples more profoundly. Psychological caretaking is not viewed by OB/Gyns as their responsibility. Women have to prepare themselves mentally for their birth since OB/Gyns do not attach much significance to mental attitude for a successful pregnancy and birth.

More women are turning to their doctors for no type of support or services other than medical delivery of their babies. During pregnancy and birth, contact with childbirth educators, labor coaches and friends are more frequent and less formal than with their doctor. Those who have an unassisted homebirth with no one else present are able to provide most of the emotional support they need. However, there are some cases where women would have done it differently, choosing to have someone in addition to their partners at their births.

A doctor who treats the woman as "matter" rather than a "mind" uses drugs, tools and technology during birth. Relieving pain through attitude, mental imagery or meditation, tinctures, herbs and other remedies is healthier, safer and as effective as drugs administered in the hospital. Most couples do not expect anything to go wrong at home even though many make arrangements for medical emergencies. It is rare that the baby's or mother's life will be in danger.

A business

Whether they operate a private practice or work for an organization, doctors are part of a business trying to make profits and avoid lawsuits. Processing customers as quickly as possible with minimal effort becomes one goal. A patient may wait for over thirty minutes in a doctor's office and the doctor breezes in and out within five minutes during a pre-natal appointment.

Women's health professionals strive for surgery, chemical dependence and intervention. If it cannot be cut, prescribed, or tampered with to facilitate a quick outcome, there may not be much incentive to offer help. There is no desire to wait on problems, wean women from chemical dependence or encourage healthier solutions. Obstetricians whose goal is to make money vie for surgeries, C-sections and the sale of contraceptive devices. They order tests and prescribe drugs from companies in which they may have stock. Any situation which can be capitalized on is fair game.

A woman enters the hospital and the *time* it takes for her to produce the child can become her greatest competitor. The countdown to birth begins and if her race with time is not sufficient according to the doctor or staff, she will be tampered with. When labor came to a halt, the doctor took my friend Janet's husband aside and explained that if things did not pick up within ten minutes, a C-section would have to be performed. Fortunately, Janet did not become one of the *failure to progress* statistics. As the doctor left the room to inform her husband, a nurse had her change positions, which was enough to stimulate the final passage of the baby.

In their haste to perform surgeries, doctors may not take much time to counsel patients. A basic medical explanation is offered to a bewildered patient who is about to undergo a permanent change. For example, a busy gynecologist informs his patient that he will have to remove a section of her vulva because of basal cell carcinoma, but he will not even tell the woman how long recovery will be, when she can resume sex or how it will affect her physically. Same thing goes for major life-changing surgeries such as tubal ligations and hyster-ectomies. If the woman does not ask obvious questions, she may not even be told key information. Doctors cannot be totally blamed for not sharing information; in their haste to service so many customers, they simply do not take the time.

One year the doctor may perform a tubal ligation. Five years later the same woman may be inquiring about a reversal. Two years later the woman may be taking fertility drugs. There is no concept of lifelong gynecological goals, but a haphazard approach to immediate whims.

If there is a psychological role that the doctor plays, it is often prompted by the need to complete paperwork. A half-hearted attempt is made when asking a woman prior to an abortion, "Are you okay with this?" During the initial pre-natal interview, many women are asked if the pregnancy was a choice. Asking if the woman is going to breastfeed or bottle-feed is another data-gathering inquiry, and that is all it often remains. Even though he may write the response "breastfeeding" on the chart, many delivery room procedures do not support the mother's choice; the baby is not immediately given to the mother to encourage breastfeeding. Many nurseries decide to bring the baby to the new mother every four hours and give him or her glucose water even though breastfeeding was annotated in the records.

A woman discovers she is pregnant and happily traipses off to her doctor. One of the first determinations a doctor makes is whether this pregnancy was a choice and if the woman is happy about it. He needs to gauge what his participation will be, whether it is abortion or birth. If the woman chooses birth, he can estimate whether the birth will involve a C-section, heavy medication or a natural birth based on her general health, attitude, appearance, past births and fear level.

When it comes time for labor and delivery, nurses monitor patients, while keeping in touch on the phone with the doctor. Many doctors arrive as late as possible for the delivery. Thousands of women do not get the doctor of their choice attending their birth, and in some cases the doctor does not even make it to the birth. He either decided he had plenty of time or had fallen back to sleep at home, and many delivery room nurses find themselves lying for a no-show doctor. Although it is not the rule, it is not uncommon for a doctor to arrive a few minutes after the birth and take credit for it. Guilt feelings will pass since the doctor has many more patients awaiting his expertise.

And how about midwives who do not make it to the homes of couples on time for the birth? Not only are couples disappointed and resentful that the attendant of their choice did not show up, but they may panic and feel unprepared. Many midwives expect their full fee whether they show up or not. Written agreements should be made when money is to be exchanged for services. Contracts enforce the notion that childbirth is first and foremost a business transaction rather than a loving, caring event.

When positive things happen in the hospital, changes come about slowly. My friend, who is an obstetrics nurse described a birth where a certified nurse-midwife learned something new. The midwife, with over twenty years experience, was amazed when she witnessed a patient deliver the baby in a squatting position. The birth was very easy and painless. Feeling excited about the possibility of the hospital implementing changes, I asked my friend if they were going to encourage women to give birth in this manner. My hopes were dashed when she said that the staff would not embrace the idea because they would not want to give up their power and control. The staff prefers to do what is most convenient for themselves.

Insurance companies versus patients

Because the doctor or hospital needs to please the insurance company rather than the patient, it is not important to be dedicated or loyal to the patient. The hospital, doctor's reputation, paycheck, and patient's insurance provider are more significant. If mistakes are made, the patient may never know it. Some explanation is offered rather than an apology or admission of error. Some doctors hope that patients will remain ignorant and not enter litigation.

Only a few courageous people demand that doctors become more responsive to customer service. It is the end user, the patient, who must become more assertive not only with their doctors, but with the insurance company. Patients would be wise to refuse medical tests, prescriptions and certain treatments that they feel are unnecessary even though costs may be fully covered by the insurance company. This takes a lot of energy on the part of patients, because they must first take the time to research and then they must assert their beliefs.

Many Americans have decided not to purchase health coverage, thereby becoming victims of the mistaken belief that they are underprivileged and need insurance. The fact is that they either (1) do not seek traditional medical solutions and will not use the coverage or (2) pay for services as needed, believing that (during the course of several years) the cost of premiums will exceed the cost of medical care for their families.

Maltreatment during pregnancy and birth

Most of the tests done during pregnancy assume the worst, but this is not surprising, since doctors are trained to detect and treat problems. While pregnant with my first child, three vials of blood were taken for routine screening. Eight years later, they needed five vials for analysis, and most of the new tests were for venereal diseases and other ailments that can be passed from a mother to baby caused by a non-monogamous relationship. It disappoints me that more women do not refuse these tests. Insurance companies fully encourage or require the tests taken during pregnancy and at birth.

We need to have a more optimistic outlook rather than assuming the worst. Risks and implications of some tests that are performed later on in the pregnancy are not truthfully conveyed, but presented so that women will submit to AFP tests, amniocentesis, CVI, ultrasound, glucose tolerance tests and blood tests. *The patient is serving the doctor so that he can effectively deliver an object of his profession (baby) in an institution (hospital) at his convenience.*

Treating the body as a machine while excluding the fact that we are complex human beings is humiliating. There were times when I had to lie still for a catheter or suppository to be inserted into my body, and I wasn't released from the hospital until my body performed certain actions. In most instances, the patient has almost no time to adjust mentally to what is going to happen. During my first birth, the doctor said he was going to "do a little cut." That episiotomy and stitching afterward hurt more than the delivery of the baby. I could hardly walk or sit comfortably for almost two weeks. I was lucky that it healed within six weeks; some women have problems for several months and even up to a year. Other women tear during birth after an episiotomy has been performed.

The pushing stage is the highlight of the birth room drama that goes on in hospitals. It marks the final scene of the pregnancy where the obstetrician can assert his authority by ordering or yelling at the mother to comply with his judgment. In many ways I was a subservient patient in my first four hospital births. I gave birth freely and consciously, but there was still a delivery involved. The first two births involved a doctor telling me when to push and how hard to push. At the next two births, they asked me to tell them when I felt like pushing. The births were easier and less painful when I was more autonomous and when the baby and I were encouraged to act instinctively.

Every day, unsuspecting mothers are violated in the delivery room. Pitocin is used to speed up births; abdomens are aggressively manipulated to extract placentas. During my fourth delivery, I was told to lie very still while the doctor inserted the internal fetal monitor. I was proud of myself for being such a cooperative patient! After the birth, I was convinced that some device the doctor used caused a small scar underneath Christina's hairline. Of course, the doctors covered for each other and no one agreed with my accusation. "It's a birthmark," they said.

Pressure

If patients do not conform to the doctor's way of doing things, they will feel subtle pressures. Women who voice opposition to blood tests, ultrasounds, the AFP test and amniocentesis are met with perplexed looks by medical practitioners, because it is hard for these workers to understand a refusal, especially if the insurance company covers the expense. They feel that all of these tests are safe and are in the best interests of the mother and child, but medical professionals often do not know the risks of some of these tests, and they do not live with the psychological dilemma women are faced with when abnormal results are revealed. The weight of an abortion decision may be placed solely on the pregnant couple. Or, the couple may worry, feel frustration, anger or grief during the remaining months of pregnancy.

Doctors in every profession make arrangements for nonconformists. I've had to sign records refusing to take the AFP test and routine ultrasounds. A dental hygienist once wrote comments in my records about my refusal to take routine bite-wing x-rays and a pediatrician annotated remarks about how he finally convinced us to give the PKU test to Millicent. All of this intolerance of patient choices has made me cut down on visits. I believe in basic care, but I do not agree with many routine procedures. If I feel it is medically necessary, I will submit to tests and immunizations.

We took our daughter to the pediatrician three days after her birth. I did not plan on immunizations and the practice "turned my name in" to the state department of health and environmental control. A few weeks later I got a certified letter signed by a doctor informing me of the dangers of not having certain tests and vaccinations. I finally decided that I did not need doctors when my family was healthy.

Cruelty

A beautiful baby is born and one of the first questions out of a doctor's mouth is "what about birth control?" Even though most of us need to consider it, this seems to be a negative question at a time when positive emotions are very high. I discontinued breastfeeding one child so that I could get back on the pill and resume some sort of "normalcy."

The influence an obstetrician has transfers to his gynecologist role with reminders that keep women in need of his services: "What type of birth control do you want? Come periodically for your pap smear and mammogram. A tubal ligation is a simple outpatient procedure."

I used to think obstetricians chose their profession, based in part, on a love for children and a desire to help women. How could I have been so naive? My doctors and the few midwives I met did not seem genuinely interested in the potential impact they have on women's lives.

The following are true examples of cruel behaviors:

(1) While in delivery, a nurse overheard the doctor making fun of his patient's weight and appearance behind the patient's back.

(2) While my doctor was performing an internal exam during my fifth pregnancy, he made some joke about a basketball team. He asked how big my house was, as if to judge whether I was economically capable of handling several children. I was not interested in this type of small-talk while in that position.

(3) Our family physician recommended that my husband undergo a vasectomy after our third child was born. "It's a very simple procedure and can be performed in the office." Sort of like a quickie divorce to rid yourself of a problem.

(4) Doctors asked if this was finally going to be "it" with the number of children we had.

(5) Some of my friends and their husbands who have had more than two children were asked by the doctor in the birth-

ing room if they wanted a tubal ligation at the time of the C-section. No discussion. No time to think it over.

(6) At the birth of my first child, I arrived at the hospital nine centimeters dilated. The nurse called the doctor and woke him up from a sound sleep. When he walked into the birthing room, he made comments about almost going off the road. It was obvious I had inconvenienced him. Later, while he was ordering me to push, he and my husband's eyes were glued to some skit from *The Late Show* on the television in the corner of the room. To spite them, I didn't push on that contraction. When he said he was going to make a small cut, I did not imagine that an episiotomy would be so painful, more than the birth itself. Before exiting, the doctor came over and said, "Have a good life" to the baby. That was the first of four hospital births characterized by insincerity and forced social politeness.

(7) During my third pregnancy, I selected a particular doctor out of three in his practice. When I called him during labor, he said he would meet me at the hospital in one hour. When I got to the hospital, I was disappointed to meet a different doctor from the practice. An effortless, painless birth occurred within ten minutes of arrival. Instead of praise, the doctor's sarcastic remark was, "I hate you!" She mentioned how her birth experience was a difficult one. I didn't need her envy at that time and I said, "Don't hate me" with the few breaths I could muster.

(8) A labor and delivery room nurse described a doctor as a monster. The OB/Gyn wanted to be on time for a musical performance. A woman's labor was not progressing as fast as the doctor wanted so a vacuum extractor was used for 45 minutes. The baby was born with respiratory problems. Meanwhile, the doctor was trying to hurry another patient in the next room.

(9) An expectant mom anticipates her first ultrasound at

twelve weeks. After eight hours of intense testing, no heart-beat is found. The doctor kept saying, "I can either do a D&C now or you'll be in the hospital in three days." This pressure made the woman visualize hemorrhaging to death if she returned home without having an immediate D&C. The doctor may have felt irresponsible if after identifying the dead baby, he let the woman return home for a natural beginning or completion of the miscarriage. After the procedure ended, the confused mother demanded to see the fetus three times until they finally showed her. Although people think they are sparing others from emotional pain by sheltering them from death, it can be more damaging to deny death.

Fertility awareness

A majority of Americans spend a large portion of their adult lives avoiding pregnancy. Professionals recommend artificial contraception, solutions which cost money, benefit someone else or keep us enslaved to a system.

Artificial contraception is a profitable business and most methods are not in the best interests of our health. As young adults become sexually active, they are not taught about their fertility—the beauty of it, what it means, and how to use it to get desired effects, whether it be avoiding or achieving pregnancy.

Many doctors believe: (1) people are unwilling to take the time and effort it requires to understand their bodies; (2) natural means of birth control requires an intelligence that most people do not have; (3) too many people make mistakes; (4) fertility is unreliable; (5) we are basically selfish; (6) there is no demand for fertility awareness.

Many employees of gynecologists claim that women want their pills and other contraceptive devices. Nobody asks about fertility awareness. That does not mean that people are knowledgeable about natural methods of birth control and have decided against it. In many cases, women do not know the techniques and benefits of natural fertility methods.

When Shannon McNear attended an initial prenatal appointment, the doctor did not understand her explanation of her fertility cycle. He insisted that ovulation occurs fourteen days after the first day of the menstrual cycle. Since he was not willing to learn the basic facts, he could not appreciate or support natural birth control methods.

Every young woman should be taught fertility awareness as part of her sex education. Accepting fertility as a beautiful gift and not a curse demonstrates appreciation. Men and women need to come to terms with their reproductive capacity, rather than try to ignore, medicate or destroy it. And that does not mean you should desire or produce several children if you are going to be irresponsible about raising them.

Respecting fertility and the natural process of childbirth can help eliminate fear and pessimism, because when you know about something, you are less apt to fear it or to be discouraged by it. Rather, you start to become self-reliant and do not need the experts (or their drugs) anymore. That is exactly why the experts do not encourage fertility awareness.

Fertility awareness and natural birth control are seldom mentioned as a solution to teen pregnancy or population control. Each political faction is looking for ways to spend money to solve the world's problems, whether it is providing artificial birth control or spending money to teach abstinence. Fertility awareness is a threat to anyone with clout because the power lies with the individual who practices the fertility awareness method.

Women are not likely to get instruction on natural means of birth control from their doctors or other women because it is not a very popular or practiced method. There are, however, organizations and resources available for those interested, and most communities have a few childbirth educators or teaching couples familiar with natural family planning (NFP).

Perhaps the most efficient way to bring about change is for mothers to educate their daughters. Women do a fabulous job of passing on information about topics such as fashion, beauty, romance, childcare, parenting, and workplace issues, but a substandard job in understanding fertility and birth.

They must know birth is intimate and sexual

Those who deliver babies on a routine basis must know that birth is an intimate, sexual affair. The childbirth industry has taken a sensual and private affair and has made it mechanical and public. This is not fair to women. In *Immaculate Deception*, Suzanne Arms describes an obstetrician who learned to deliver women who were

> ...shaved, draped and on their backs.... Male physicians may have felt more comfortable with the woman well covered and with her body distorted by forceps, spinals, tons of drugs. Then they did not have to think of the sexual implications of their work. Observing denuded parts, vulva and vagina only, they could lead themselves to think they were working on a 'machine.' (Rothman 1982: 182)

Doctors feel uncomfortable around a laboring woman. They focus their attention on all the mechanical devices in the room—the monitors, the IV. How much eye to eye contact is made between the doctor and patient during the final moments of birth? Probably not a whole lot. The doctor avoids it because it is uncomfortable. It is uncomfortable because it is private, sensual and sexual. Many doctors leave laboring women in the room with other female nurses to avoid social discomfort. They appear when birth is imminent.

A woman feels a certain awe for her doctor after he delivers the baby. After all, they shared one of the most significant personal moments in the woman's life. I can remember details of my birth experiences, even the name and general appearance of the intern who performed the D&C on me after a miscarriage over ten years ago. Most women can recall their birth experiences with little or no effort. Doctors must know that patients form attachments with them. Many offices proudly display large photo albums containing pictures, cards and letters from new mothers. Most of these letters perceive the doctor as a hero and are full of admiration.

When describing the birth of her forty year-old son, my aunt recalls the doctor saying they should be on a first name basis after her natural, unmedicated delivery. This was the doctor's first experience with a patient opting for no medication and was a very bold act during the late 1950's. Both the doctor and Aunt Jeri shared a moment which was far from a medical procedure.

Secrets your doctor will never tell you

There are many secrets obstetricians will not tell you. Some possibilities as to why: (1) the doctor acts in ways that will justify the need for his expertise; (2) the doctor wants to put his medical training to use; (3) impatience; (4) disinterest; (5) it is not his responsibility to tell you every detail or secret for success; (6) he may not know some secrets that will benefit you.

Secrets you need to know:

- There is a high error rate in many of the prenatal tests.
- Strengthen your perineum for birth (which would decrease the likelihood of an episiotomy or tears. During pregnancy: Kegel exercises, perineal massage, squatting and tailor-sitting exercises will practically eliminate the need for an episiotomy. During birth: Applying warm compresses to the perineum and delivering in a squatting or standing position will also help. Do not hurry the birth or be overly aggressive about pushing. Patience is important.
- Mental readiness is extremely important for birth.
- Major decisions are based on inaccurate technology. For example, a C-section might be performed because

the EFM indicated that the baby was in distress: his heart rate stopped. For a split-second, all babies heart rates stop as they are ready to be born.
- There are risks and effects of legal drugs used during labor.
- The brain-body connection at birth should not be tampered with.
- Every birth could culminate in an orgasm.
- Birth is a straightforward, uncomplicated process. Labor may be lengthy and some doctors are bored with uncomplicated deliveries.
- You (and your baby) are not totally safe in the hospital. There is a risk of contracting a staphylococcus infection.
- Your doctor may be unfit to attend a perfectly normal, natural birth. His training, ego and temperament are suited for problems, surgery and abnormality.
- A C-section is major surgery and should be avoided. Your doctor probably won't go out of his way to help you avoid a C-section.
- Doctors will not tell you how to have a successful birth experience.

Three phrases a doctor will never say to a patient: "I made a mistake." "I was wrong." "I'm sorry."

Three things a patient will never tell her doctor: "I'm smarter than you think." "I don't need you as much as you think I do. In fact, you need me more than I need you." "You're not a god. You simply chose your profession and pursued it. I admire you for that, but I do not worship you."

Unassisted birthers favorite secrets

Many women who have had unassisted homebirths are childbirth educators or have studied midwifery. Their wisdom can be helpful to any woman who is pregnant. As with any suggestion, individuals vary in their responses and preferences. For example, blue cohosh may help speed up labor, but can have dangerous effects on some women if taken at the wrong time. Castor oil may help, but it makes many women sick. Staying on your feet during labor may be helpful, but many women find that moving around during labor can be disruptive to concentration. Textbooks claim that squatting is the best position for birth, but I was extremely uncomfortable when I tried squatting. I preferred a supported-kneeling position for delivery.

What can you share about pregnancy and delivery that we don't often find written about?

It is not essential to know how far dilated you are at any stage of labor. We tried checking once and weren't sure of the results, but it didn't matter—the baby came anyway!

Episiotomies and tears are not inevitable. Both of my daughters were over 8 lbs. and were born over an intact perineum. Soaking in a tub, hot compresses, Kegels and perineal massage help.

Toxemia is completely preventable through a proper diet. Good protein, salt and fluid intake are essential.

Having the cord around the baby's neck is not necessarily an emergency requiring clamping and cutting. Corrine's cord was wrapped twice around her neck and my husband simply unlooped it....It is also unnecessary and harmful to clamp and cut the cord before it stops pulsing. We didn't cut the cord until the placenta was out and then we didn't even clamp it. Not clamping helps reduce jaundice and sometimes you can use the cord blood that escapes for blood typing or PKU.

As much as they love to, never let your doctor induce. My doctor wanted to induce my labor before my due date because I was three centimeters dilated for quite some time. He was afraid I'd have the baby in the car. Little did he know that I planned a homebirth with a midwife. Later in my pediatrician's office, I spoke to two women who happen to have the same OB as I do. Both their labors were induced and both their babies were early.

Induced labor is harder and riskier for the mother and baby. Breaking water does not start labor or speed it up in most cases.

Epidurals are not safe. They do carry risks.

I would recommend both partners memorizing scripture pertaining to childbirth, taking liquid calcium and listening to peaceful music during labor.

Stay on your feet when in labor. Walk faster and breathe slower with each contraction. Rather than thinking, "Oh no, here comes a contraction," think ,"Oh, yes! A good strong one; that's what I want."

Stay on your feet, still, when pushing. Don't push. Your baby will move down. You open the door and let her out.

Upright position during labor and birth, such as squatting and kneeling, assists birth and prevents tearing or need for episiotomy.

Movement is good for the laboring mother and standing is a good and safe way to deliver your child.

Nipple stimulation is an effective means of inducing labor. My pregnancies have all been over 41 weeks gestation and two have been almost 43 weeks. I read about nipple stimulation in a few midwifery publications, but there were no instructions on how to do it. I used it to induce labor the last two times. It should not be tried until at least 38 weeks gestation, as it could cause premature labor. You can start or speed up labor by doing it properly.

High protein and complete diet will decrease chances of complicated pregnancy or birth. No weight restrictions and salt food to taste.... There are breech position exercises and herbs / homeopathics to turn a breech presentation. It's better than a C-section.... Uninterrupted bonding after the birth and rooming-in will help establish a sound breastfeeding relationship.

For Rh negative mothers who choose not to have Rhogam: the baby's blood will seldom mix with the mother's unless there is trauma to the placenta, or if the placenta is not allowed to detach itself naturally in its own time, like when the cord is pulled on.

Even more important than nutrition or exercise is one's frame of mind, trust in oneself and knowledge of modern medicine and allopathic practices. It's important that you know what you do not want. In the beginning of three of my labors, I took black and blue cohosh. It helped speed the process immediately. Cayenne pepper stops hemorrhaging. Bach flower remedies help husband to focus on labor and not fear. Goldenseal and tea trea oil get rid of infection after labor on cord clamp and can help women internally. Chlorophyll and Alfalfa and Spirulina build women's energy back up. V-C 10.000 units and breastfeeding helps baby's immunity against infection. Apply papaya slices on tears after birth. Comfrey on tears will help to heal. Homeopathic emergency kit should be on hand at all times.

For pregnancy: Guave leaves are very effective against nausea in pregnancy. Take Spirulina every day. B-12 and protein are very important. Alfalfa has 92 minerals in it and is high in iron and also constipates. Visualization of love power of female respect and honor of birthing women. Ritual visualization of father as part creator of the child and not solely a money-maker in the family.

You *relax* when your husband is between your legs. You *tense* up when anyone else is there whether it is your doctor, midwife or your own mother. You need privacy.

Holding your own hot, throbbing flesh-of-my-flesh as it leaves your body is very sensuous. Why do you think they wear gloves?

Doctor intervention leads to more intervention. Birth is a simple and natural process.

Why your doctor doesn't want you too knowledgeable

Your doctor does not want you to know too much because your knowledge may thwart his goals, making you a disruption to the system in place. His training and approach may be different from your ideas, and his ego and expertise may be challenged if you know more than he does. Besides, his business is threatened if you discover you do not need him.

Women who know too much are often treated with condescension, and labor coaches or doulas frequently encounter hostility. They are often ridiculed because, while the nurses prefer the woman to stare at an object on the wall and do mindless breathing exercises, the labor coach has other methods to benefit the laboring mom.

A friend of mine volunteered at a home for unwed teens. She assisted them during their pregnancies and births. During one of her first births, she was trying to encourage the mother, yet being careful to remain neutral so that the teen could make decisions about her labor and birth. The certified nurse-midwife who delivered the child said to my friend, "What have you been reading, Nature Woman? *Spiritual Midwifery?*" My friend was scolded for interfering with the patient's desire (and staff's pressure) to have a drugged childbirth. Neither the home for unwed teens nor the hospital appreciated my friend's help, so she ended up quitting soon afterward.

The greatest obstacle to discovery is not ignorance—it is the illusion of knowledge. —Daniel J. Boorstin

Husband and wife giving birth privately in their own home—this is a very important aspect of marriage that we are introducing to the public, one that many people would rather we not speak about. But it must be done. The medical model of birth undermines the marriage promises made the day the couple was wed. —Marilyn Moran

13

Healing Wounds

Act of Love:
O My God, I love Thee above all things with my whole heart and soul, because Thou are all good and deserving of all my love. I love my neighbor as myself for the love of Thee. I forgive all who have injured me and ask pardon of all whom I have injured. Amen.

Discovery, shock and denial

Discovering that birth was a sensual, even sexual experience triggered anger. I was angry because my past births needed healing. I was upset that millions of women will never experience sensual births because of the limitations and hindrances placed upon them at birth. During my fifth pregnancy I asked myself, "Why didn't anyone tell me what birth was all about?" and "Why hadn't I realized that I could have pursued childbirth outside a hospital?"

It was hard to admit that I prostituted myself to a system filled with people who do not genuinely care. The anger I felt about my experiences expanded into anger that other women submit to similar childbirth practices, and I began to grieve about the whole approach to childbirth in this country. Every day, thousands of women are subjected to needless monitoring, amniotomies, inductions, episiotomies, epidurals and delivery in an uncomfortable position. Their pain, fear and negative attitude about birth contributes to an avoidance rather than a celebration of the process.

When we do not research all of the alternatives, we end up complying with the most widely practiced approach. I dutifully attended all of my prenatal appointments and after birth, took my children to all of their well-child visits with a family physician or pediatrician. Very rarely did I have concerns or problems with the health of myself or my family. I was proud of myself for ensuring they got all of their immunizations.

Then I had my fifth child. Not only did I not waste my time going back and forth to doctors, we decided not to immunize. One major reason we researched immunizations is that we encountered families whose children had died as a direct result of immunizations. We also learned that many seizures and disabilities are caused by immunizing healthy children, and that a society's immune system is radically altered (and not necessarily for the best) when the healthy masses are immunized. Brochures picturing deathly ill children encourage parents to immunize against measles, whooping cough and chickenpox. I no longer believe that failing to immunize against certain childhood diseases will cause death, mental illness or physical handicaps if a child should contract one of these illnesses. I now see the propaganda with a whole new perspective and I feel sorry for parents who do not know the risks or actual benefits of each immunization.

Had I been given an opportunity to make different decisions with my older four, I would have chosen to reduce my number of visits with doctors during times of wellness. Now I am more informed about pregnancy, birth and childcare based on written research, confidence, and networking with other knowledgeable women. My baby is healthy and I am much happier without any interfering opinions, judgment or "permission" to raise my children.

We should not criticize our past mistakes and choices. Although I would love to go back and make changes in my birth experiences, I had one hospital birth that was very pleasant and three that were generally satisfying. Those births were not as intrinsically rewarding as our unassisted homebirth, but it does not mean that the other children are less loved or insignificant compared to our youngest. In fact, a greater love has blossomed within our family. Since our unassisted homebirth, I have felt an endless supply of love that I am able to share with other children, friends and anyone who is receptive. I did not feel that way after my first four births.

The childbirth scam

It was not until we had our daughter at home that we realized what a scam the whole childbirth industry is. Most women and their babies would do fine with only a fraction of the medical care given. Unfortunately, the more strongly one clings to the childbirth myths and the less confident women are in their ability to have a baby, the more likely they will seek experts to deliver their child. The experts are not willing to give up their positions and want us to believe that we are lost without them. We must never blindly accept the idea that doctors, midwives, childbirth educators or well-respected friends are some type of omniscient and omnipotent god. They are fallible human beings and are not immune to life's struggles. Doctors have simply chosen a profession and all we can do is trust their competence and judgment. It is very tempting for doctors, or any professional, to abuse their position by encouraging patients to idolize them.

It is flattering to be perceived as a god, and it takes humility to convince others to lower their opinions. The god-like doctor has the power to control events. His freedom goes unquestioned as he induces a woman simply because another patient will soon deliver in the next room. It would be very convenient to complete his deliveries in order to be on time for a social function or to go home to sleep. The ultimate

---

In our culture, doctors are allowed to inflict pain on babies and children. No parent would allow anyone else to do this. We must begin to respect babies and children's physical/emotional boundaries. -Valarie Nordstrom

control is to ensure that most babies are born during convenient working hours.

Episiotomies, amniotomies, epidurals, C-sections, routine ultrasound and prenatal tests are part of having babies. Many of these procedures go unquestioned while the patient allows the doctor to make major decisions. Women are told what to do and how to behave during childbirth when they attend hospital-sponsored classes. With the money that is involved in the childbirth industry, very few people or organizations who make a living from childbirth are willing to see changes. The only change they want to see is an increase in customers.

Customers do not demand clear or strict standards from the medical professionals and facilities. Because they have followed society's customs for pregnancy, patients' goals are often similar to doctors' goals.

What birth wounds do we need to heal?

- our own personal birth wounds
- the wounds of friends, family and other women
- the anger and sadness that up to 25% of all babies in this country are born via C-section. David Stewart, Executive Director of the International Association of Parents and Professionals for Safe Alternatives in Childbirth, says that six of seven C-sections are medically unnecessary and that a practitioner's C-section rate should be less than 5%
- the realization that some women do not care that they fall in the lowest part of *The Birth Pyramid*
- a cultural birth system that is not in the best interests of those it serves
- the prevalence of the myths of birth
- the realization that there is an abundance of conforming (non-thinking, unquestioning) people in our culture
- the very powerful opposition to alternative birth, opposition so strong that many people do not attempt

better births
- the psychological discomfort we feel for others. Men and women will be having dissatisfying births today, tomorrow and for years to come

The grieving process and how we can heal our wounds

Each person progresses through the healing process at his own pace. The deeper the wound, the more challenging the healing process. The greater the expectations, the greater the possibility for disappointment. The grieving process not only applies to death, but to any loss. Many women and men do not feel a sense of completeness or fulfillment at birth and are instead upset about their birth events. It may take them some time to mentally recover from an unnecessary C-section or early induction which produced a premature baby.

The grieving process may leave you restless or exhausted, or you may have trouble eating or sleeping. Stages overlap and anger may emerge at any time and even those who feel they are completely recovered often discover more anger. The intensity of emotions varies from person to person. As a result, not everyone progresses smoothly from grief, through anger and pain, to acceptance. Some remain stuck on one stage for many months, while others complete the entire process in less than a year.

(1) Grief

Grief is a normal and painful emotional response to a loss. It is a state of mind and body, often a lonely process where we must learn to tolerate loss and construct new ways of living or thinking about the past. The event itself may not have been monumental, but the significance placed on the loss will effect the ability to move forward. I know a woman who desired a perfect birth and when it fell short of perfection, marital difficulties increased. She resented her husband, who did not meet her expectations. Another woman despised her two birth experiences so much that she did not go through childbirth again. She was heavily drugged during the C-sections and saw one baby several hours later, after relatives and others touched and held her baby first.

Early stages of grief may bring about panic and fear as we try to link our past with our future. As we come to tolerate our loss we can look towards the future with greater self-knowledge and inner strength, gaining knowledge to help ourselves or others, giving us hope, and helping us cope with our losses.

The grieving process involves a combination of the following: denial, isolation, anger, frustration, resentment, bargaining, depression, guilt, remorse, acceptance and hope. Grief can involve intense mental anguish or deep sorrow. After I decided that childbirth is a scam and a multi-billion dollar industry concerned more with money than with the people it serves, I had to work through intense mental anguish and sorrow over the way birth generally occurs in our society. One reason many women do not want several children is because they dread childbirth, having been convinced that pregnancy is uncomfortable and unattractive, and birth is an ordeal that the doctor helps you through.

I do not feel excited about the way newborns are welcomed into the world. We can only hope that men and women will gain the courage and strength to make bold choices, leading to a time when women trust themselves more than they trust their doctors. But for the time being, women seem to accept that we go to doctors who deliver babies in hospitals.

(2) Anger

After recovering from the initial shock and denial, it is common to feel anger, resentment, envy or rage. Blaming others is a common part of anger.

I encounter people on a weekly basis whose birth stories contain some atrocity, injustice or flagrant disregard for womanhood. Just because these women do not define their births as dissatisfying does not mean everything is okay; they are being violated unknowingly. The source of my anger is directed towards (1) the medical profession, (2) a culture that devalues motherhood, and (3) women, for submitting to current pregnancy and birth practices.

I have heard many accounts of C-sections that occurred because labor would not progress or because the mother was afraid and persuaded the doctor to schedule a repeat C-section. Most people know someone whose baby was in distress because the EFM indicated that the heartbeat had stopped momentarily. Since labor was not progressing even after drugs were administered to augment labor, an emergency C-section was performed. I have known women to be induced simply because they went past an estimated due date and others induced only to bear a premature child. This is insane and the only way the insanity will be stopped is when all women take charge during their pregnancies and births. Refusing tests, demanding natural childbirth, allowing no one to pressure them into a decision with which they are uncomfortable. Take time to think about what is best for you and your baby.

But many women not wanting to take charge of their own births, comply with tests and the implementation of technology, believing that the doctor will make appropriate decisions. The grief process begins when women realize that they gave too much power to the doctor and did not take enough responsibility in decision-making. Anger, guilt and blame all occur simultaneously, paving the way for depression and despair.

Anger serves a useful purpose when it is applied in a positive manner or leads to maturity, but anger is destructive when it is based on faulty assumptions. Assuming that a doctor is malicious and incompetent does you no good if he is genuinely trying to protect women from pain, fear, and death.

Elisabeth Kübler-Ross, author of *On Death and Dying* stated that fear, guilt and loneliness are part of the anger process. It is normal to feel rage and injustice. She believes that sharing feelings with others is therapeutic. When we can face the fear, hurt, guilt and helplessness, our anger often lessens.

The passage of time can help. When we fear, we have a problem with trust. It takes time to rebuild our optimism and trust in others. Guilt is experienced when we feel that not enough was said or done to prevent an occurrence. Guilt after an unpleasurable birth is usually directed at ourselves rather than the doctor.

Anger is often the result of sadness, fear, insecurity, help-lessness, powerlessness, disappointment, unmet expectations or unfulfilled dreams. It may be the result of the need for love, care, respect or acknowledgment. Anger is usually a temporary reaction to feeling threatened. Anger that is not effectively dealt with will turn to resentment, making forgive-ness unlikely. Anger may then reside in someone's heart in the form of chronic resentment and pessimism. We cannot move forward when we are trapped in resentment, judgment or name-calling. Suffering and forgiveness take a lot of ac-tive work, and the feelings behind the anger need to be chan-neled in positive directions.

(3) Pain and disappointment, depression and despair

Those who have had unassisted homebirths may not have started out on the top of *The Birth Pyramid.* They usually have had births which were less than ideal. Just because a couple may have had a private birth does not mean it was necessarily a perfect birth. When aspirations are beyond what we can touch, feel and see, it is easy to despair if the goal is not attained. Childbirth is an opportunity to experience the infinite, but when it is not done in privacy, it is difficult to achieve the infinite.

As the grieving person moves beyond anger, it is not un-common for sorrow and despair to set in, causing us to yearn for what we have lost and take little pleasure in what we have. Women realize that they will give birth only a few times during their lives and that there is no way to replace a birth event, leading many women to struggle to accept what happened at their previous births. Some may not even be able to endure the memory of their births and may describe them as more pleasant than they actually were. There is still pain and despair that has not been reconciled with. Most women strive to make improvements on their next pregnancies and births, while some are compelled to help others avoid elements from their birth encounters.

Many happy families who have had private births have been dismissed as eccentric and irresponsible. When cultural forces are brought to bear against this minority, they often form a network as a way of sharing their pain. Bureaucrats may make it difficult to obtain a birth certificate and doctors may refuse to examine a mother in need of medical expertise. Fortunately, the same tenacious people who carried out alternative birth plans also have the characteristics necessary to gain strength.

Emotional pain manifests itself in physical ways, such as overeating, lost sleep, constricted muscles, breathing trouble or high blood pressure. Our pain can keep our hearts closed and separate from others. If we continue to blame or judge others, we have decided to remain incapacitated. We may pity ourselves, feel unworthy or act superior. The pain we feel needs to be expressed in a safe, secure place. When we can let go of pain, we can begin to heal by making room for kindness, love and compassion. It is like letting go of a final burden. Despair disappears when there is a strong basis for hope.

When I think about how babies are born in this country, I feel pain more than resentment, anger, fear or frustration. Pain because many people have passively accepted the way we do business in having babies. It is painful to know that thousands of men and women will be cheated each day from having an experience that could strengthen their sense of femininity, masculinity and their marriage. They will be betrayed by the system whose priorities are power, money and control. Their parenting experience will begin with a relief that the pregnancy has ended in a safe birth with a "healthy" child. It does not begin with a high level of confidence, but trepidation and insecurity, especially if it is their first child.

(4) Acceptance

Acceptance means acknowledging the abuse that goes on in maternity wings of hospitals and other emotional pain related to birth. We are neither angry nor depressed. We are not apathetic, but having come to view our experiences more objectively, the struggle is over. We often emerge more resilient and stronger, in a position to help others reach higher levels on *The Birth Pyramid*. When we go beyond sorrow, fear and anger, we expand our capacity to love and feel empathy.

Ignorance is not bliss

Knowledge enables us to make more decisions and to climb higher on *The Birth Pyramid*. Having more decisions to make may cause more stress, but it is a challenge we are faced with because we have the ability to reason. We are not better off not knowing something. Were you ever upset about learning something so late in life, after an event took place? You would have given anything to know more so that you could have made different choices. "If only I had known that!" Growth is less likely when we are uninformed.

Coping strategies

The grieving process enables us to rebuild our lives and work for something we believe in. Here are some ways to help ease the pain of grief:

- accept and express your feelings; share them with others
- cry. Crying will cleanse you
- join a support group. Form a new one if necessary

> The yearning within man for truth and love and beauty and perfection indicates that something is lacking for the fullness of life. - Fulton Sheen

- do something enjoyable
- pray, meditate, spend time in silence
- serve others or volunteer
- maintain a routine structure in your life. While grieving, life seems to be in disarray and it's easier if you do not have other complexities in life or have to think about so much
- take care of your body. Direct energy towards positive outlets
- practice forgiveness of yourself and others
- vow to improve upon your future birth experiences
- accept failings and past experiences
- focus on happy moments of past births. Exaggerate the positive and disregard painful memories
- help others to birth with joy
- help others to avoid mistakes by talking about your past births
- admit that you cannot change your birth experience, but that you have many years left to make a vital impact as a parent

Applying these ideas to your life will help you to regain enthusiasm which will help heal your birth wounds.

Forgiveness

Equally important in healing birth wounds is the capacity to forgive. Forgiveness is part of acceptance and the key to coping. If we cannot forgive ourselves and others, we remain limited and insecure. We do not need to express forgiveness outwardly in order to heal. "Forgiveness requires only a shift in perception, another way of looking at the people and circumstances that we feel have caused us upset and pain." (Casarjian 1992: 14)

The act of forgiveness poses many challenges. We may think a person or institution does not deserve our forgiveness. If we cannot forgive an obstetrician, hospital or midwife, we will be expending valuable energy. A true release will not be possible. We have the power to decide whether we will forgive. Forgiveness is a continuous process and a way of life.

If you feel angry, resentful or guilty when you think of certain people, you have not healed your wounds. You are locked in self-protection and are not enjoying optimal emotional health. Unloving thoughts and attitudes will have an effect on your body. The goal is to become your own best friend and free yourself of pain and suffering.

Doctors, midwives and people in any profession have an attachment to results. Some may not want to relinquish control and some may not be very helpful or competent. People are motivated by different forces and have limitations which they are not likely to admit. If we believe our doctor has god-like qualities, we are apt to feel discouraged when our outcomes do not meet with perfection. We may assume that secrecy, miscommunication and arrogance characterize his behavior. We do not consider the fact that doctors make mistakes.

Doctors who present themselves as a god will exhibit arrogance and withhold information, but we still need to try to forgive them. When we view them as people with vulnerabilities, we notice that they may be private, insecure people who harbor feelings of inadequacy and incompetence from time to time. When we understand that they too are human, we can forgive them more easily. Whether they have malicious intent or pure motives is not the point. We need to surrender ourselves to forgive so that we gain new insights rather than exhaust our mental resources.

The road to healing our birth wounds may be long and rocky, but we need to begin our journey so that we can mature. Our struggles and pain may intensify along the way so we must choose whether we want to live trapped in denial and disappointment or move towards acceptance and action.

> The underlying and often unconscious beliefs that we hold about ourselves and human nature influence and ultimately determine our ability and willingness to risk, to trust, to love, and to forgive. - Robin Casarjian

14

Death and Disillusion

Unassisted Homebirth Gone Awry

Unattended homebirths, like hospital deliveries, are not always perfect. Although I have heard of only one death during a DIY birth after 1990, there have been other difficulties. Babies born with meconium, in the amniotic sac, breech, and with the cord wrapped around their necks have posed no problems at DIY births. Also, some babies born as early as 36 weeks and as late as 43 weeks gestation have required no extraordinary measures. Generally, what the hospital diagnoses as troublesome is not defined as problematic at home. No one whisks the baby away to an intensive care nursery for testing and observation. Rather, the new moms cuddle their babies and continuously nurse them in the comforts of their own home. Mothers and their babies most often thrive in the absence of medical assistance.

Some of the trouble surrounding unassisted homebirths stems from marital conflicts. For example, wives may be disappointed at the lack of their husbands' enthusiasm or preparation for the upcoming birth. Also, when expectations and reality differ, there may be a secret longing on the part of the wives to have attained a more "perfect" birth.

An infant's health may be poor whether it is born at home or in the hospital. Since people believe that human error is negligible in the hospital and prominent at home, experts (doctors) are seldom questioned while amateurs (DIY couples) are almost always scrutinized.

A common problem at unassisted homebirths is the presence of the wrong people. The stories in this chapter convey the struggles and sadness that sometimes accompanies childbirth. The stories are true, but the names have been changed to maintain privacy.

Marital conflicts

Birth disappointments occur when the couple is having difficulty communicating or is experiencing marital problems. Ceceilia, a mother of three young children was expecting her fourth baby. During her pregnancy, she discovered that her husband was having an affair and had had numerous affairs throughout their marriage. She was shocked after discovering the infidelity and became emotionally exhausted, knowing that her marriage needed a lot of work. Her husband was not enthusiastic about an unassisted homebirth, and she did not know how she would go through with the unassisted birth. But, during the last few weeks of pregnancy, she and her husband began working on their problems and the birth went well.

In another situation, Juliet continued to resent her husband a year after her baby was born. Greg had not lived up to Juliet's expectations during the pregnancy or birth, nor was he interested in reading, watching videos, learning about childbirth, or attending any classes. He felt that he would simply know what to do instinctively at the moment of birth and would take cues from Juliet. Juliet had a midwife-attended homebirth and a DIY previously, but this would be her current husband's first birth experience.

Greg built a tub for a waterbirth and when Juliet entered the early stages of labor she hopped in her bathtub and asked Greg to fill the tub, but Greg saw that Juliet was comfortable, so he never bothered to fill their birthing tub. Their baby was born in the bathtub. Juliet was disappointed that Greg was not sensitive and tender enough during active labor; he was so nervous that he vomited several times. After the birth Greg confided that he did not feel the need to practice or prepare; he would be ready to handle the birth. He believed his participation in their son's birth was fine, while Juliet had a lot of anger to work through.

Cassandra and Tim's first birth was an unplanned DIY in the front seat of their car on a dark, cold night in the Alaskan wilderness. You would think he might entertain the idea of a planned DIY the next time. Not at all. Cassandra remembers arguing with her husband about having a DIY birth. "He threatened to call the police, ambulance and fire department on me if I went through with my plans! He did not agree to the homebirth until two weeks before my due date, which also happened to be the day our son was born." She went into labor and woke Tim up when birth was imminent—twenty minutes before the baby was born. Tim was afraid someone would die during birth, that social services would take away their children, or that they would get arrested. Cassandra's pregnancy was marked by anxiety as she tried to persuade and console her husband in regard to her desire for an unassisted homebirth. He finally changed his mind when he saw his wife's determination.

Another situation arose where the expectant mother desired a DIY birth and the husband was not comfortable with the idea. Their second birth was with a midwife and Marisa knew they could handle an unassisted homebirth. Dan was never fully convinced, but agreed to it anyway. As Marisa's faith increased, she began to wean herself and her family away from traditional medical care. The birth went well and the couple settled in with their new baby. But then, after two days, the baby suddenly turned blue and they rushed him to the hospital. Marisa and Dan discovered that their son had a congenital heart malfunction and would have to undergo surgery. The baby is now two years old and consumes a lot of the family's energy. Marisa and Dan now feel that they cannot handle any more children.

Marisa admits that she would never go through with a DIY again because it caused marital tensions after their son began his journey through the medical labyrinth. If there are any future pregnancies, she will have a medically trained specialist at her birth and take the baby for a thorough exam following the birth. For a short while, they had to work through resentments and self-blame, but they are healing their wounds.

Baby not breathing

Susan's prenatal care was more extensive than almost any other woman I have known. She visited a chiropractor where she had mineral wraps, adjustments, and nutritional support. Her daily routine included a bath, massage, sunbath, body brushing, reflexology, stretching, shakes and protein. She was a strict vegan for half of her pregnancy and did aerobics twice a week. She did transformational breathwork, art therapy and a few Reiki sessions. She was part of a birth support group in which the other members gave her gifts of service rather than material goods. Foot massage, tummy massage, kind words and well wishes for the baby were bestowed upon her. She spent a lot of time praying, meditating, visualizing and reading birth books. Susan had two acupuncture treatments to stimulate labor since she estimated that she was four weeks overdue.

Susan's labor was welcomed with the thought that she would not have to endure unnecessary exams, machines, fear and noise.

> As my contractions began to get intense and fast, I began to use the transformational breathwork with loud vocalization. I felt that all of my Yoga training, relaxation practice, meditation, movement, music skills, singing skills, and dancing skills had prepared me for just this moment. Time stopped and eternity was staring me right in the face. I moved from my bedroom to the bathroom as I felt inspired and motivated to do different things (dance, bathe, shower) moment by moment. While in the tub at one point I had

the fleeting thought, "I'm not sure I can do this." I could be pushing soon and I was.

When I felt completely open I decided to squat. I immediately felt Andrew rush down the birth canal and crown. My husband Jim calmly said, "That's a head!" I asked him to check for the cord, to see if it was around Andrew's neck. "No, but he looks funny," Jim replied. "I know what it is—the amniotic sac hasn't broken yet." With the next contraction, after five minutes of patient waiting, I felt like standing up in a half squat. Then we waited for five more minutes and I felt like dropping down on all fours. Jim caught him in a rush of blood and fluid.

I felt this incredible wet emptiness and my peace soon turned to panic as I watched our son lay there quietly like he was asleep. He was completely still, pink, and not breathing—no movement, nothing. I gently began to puff into his mouth. I'll never forget the feeling of my lips on his for the first time, gently puffing, but no response. I did a finger swipe and turned him over on my leg and tried to do a little heimlich maneuver. I handed him to Jim, who gave him a quick father's blessing while I prayed silently. I looked down and noticed that the cord had broken. It was purple and paper thin, but no blood was gushing out of either end, like I had read about, but I was concerned because I knew he was not getting any oxygen from my placenta.

Jim called 911 and a volunteer firefighter, who lived a few streets away, was knocking on our door within two minutes. He later told me that he knew exactly what to do when he saw Andrew. He put his mouth on my son's, sucked, then spit and gave him three quick puffs. Andrew opened his eyes, started to breathe and the volunteer passed him to the paramedics, who had just arrived. He was airlifted to the ICU, where he spent three days.

Meanwhile, I was hemorrhaging my life away and spent one hour in complete fear and panic. I would have died if my doctor didn't show up to remind someone to check my hematocrit (it was 4). He stopped the hemorrhage with pitocin and ordered me some blood. I was separated from my son for 28 hours and after three days, we came home to recover.

I have no regrets about the DIY birth. I feel nothing but happiness and peace in my heart right now. I'm so grateful for the privilege of being a mother to these beautiful souls. I feel a sense of contentment and wonder that I did this pregnancy and birth with no allopathic prenatal care. I built this 11 lb., 12 oz., 23 inch baby boy with knowledge, faith and love and I birthed him in 3-1/2 hours with no perineal damage and no pain. It is the truth. I had a painless birth. The sense of joy and contentment this brings is almost holy!

I don't know why we went through those three days of trauma, but I do know that we are protected, and we have recovered and are stronger for the experience. I wish Jim or I could have been the one who sucked him out and then spit. For whatever reason, it was not meant to be.

Shoulder dystocia

Jolie wanted her birth videotaped and enjoyed having several friends at her home during labor. When it came time for the birth and she began pushing the baby out, it seemed to get stuck. For three or four minutes, nothing happened. Then a friend of hers who had a DIY birth realized that she needed to move into another position. Jolie was in a kneeling position on the bed and was helped to a standing position where the baby freed itself. Jolie was silently praying that the baby would come out and at the moment of birth, she felt as if an angel's wings were unfolding and entering the world.

Another couple was not so fortunate. Although they had talked to midwives and read several books on nutrition, midwifery, DIY birth, labor and newborn care, they were not prepared for their baby's death.

Our daughter was stillborn at home. My husband and I had a very hard birth as my little girl weighed 10 lbs. 15 oz. She died from shoulder dystocia. Had we been in a hospital, there is the possibility that a C-section would have saved her life. We have to live with our decision now and it is very difficult to look at homebirth through the eyes of grief. Had we had someone who could have palpated and had we been able to get a good midwife or doctor, we probably wouldn't have done it alone.

My husband is guilt ridden and has no confidence to even think about helping me birth another baby. I don't know where the balance is, especially in our lives, but I'm not sure if I support homebirth with or without attendants. I hate all the unnecessary procedures which go with hospital birth, but not being able to help my suffocating baby was unbearable and I would rather go through hell than see my baby die any day of the week.

I don't think everyone is right for a homebirth in every situation and, unfortunately, I've learned that through a very painful experience. Sometimes life is a cruel teacher and this has been a very difficult lesson. Life, and sometimes babies, are fragile and statistics don't mean a thing when you are watching your baby be buried.

Unwanted guests

Cathy and Jordan told their aspiring midwife friend, Lua, that she could observe their birth. Jordan thought they would be getting some additional help and friendship. Cathy preferred a quiet, peaceful labor and called Lua minutes before the baby's birth. Lua's excitement was based on the fact that she was at a birth for personal reasons rather than to provide support. This was Cathy's fourth homebirth, so she was familiar with bearing children. When she announced that she was ready to push, Lua yelled, "No!" Lua had some fears that she brought to this birth based on problems at other births. After the baby was born, Cathy was bleeding more than normal. Lua thought that her uterus was big and insisted that she try to urinate. Cathy got up off the bed a little too quickly and as she went into the bathroom, she fainted and hit her head on the wall.

When she awoke, Lua was massaging her fundus in a panic to the point of almost rubbing her uterus out. Cathy could feel her cervix at the opening of her vagina. Cathy pushed it back and continued to rub the fundus, while blocking the uterus in place with a hand over her pubic bone. Cathy worried about whether she was all right or not. She was so exhausted and had never been at a birth where there was fear. The uterus healed and she did not hemorrhage.

Whether a woman has a child at home or in the hospital, she should understand that death, disappointment and despair can happen anywhere at anytime; it is part of life. No one place or person can protect another from the heartaches of life. We can only prepare for success and accept the end result.

PART IV

"Women's Issues"

15

Midwives' Role In The Birth Process

When I first started researching unassisted birth, I came across very little discussion dealing with why anyone would not consider having a midwife at their birth. What was lacking with midwife-attended births? Some women choose an obstetrician for their first birth, a midwife for their second and then go on to have an unassisted birth.

I decided to include a brief discussion of midwifery in this book to aid you in your decision about whether to birth alone or with an attendant. For the purpose of this discussion, I will not distinguish between certified nurse-midwife, lay midwife and direct-entry midwife, nor will I cover the legalities of midwifery. Midwives are those who have childbirth skills and serve as birth attendants.

Ask someone what they think of modern day midwives and you will undoubtedly get various responses, because a large portion of the population is not sure what midwives do and some wonder if they serve a valuable purpose. Also, many question their credentials and wonder why a consumer would select a midwife over a doctor.

Still others view midwives as "birth goddesses" and would not choose an OB/Gyn as their birth attendant. They believe that midwives are educators, advisors, friends, supporters and experts. Midwives who attend homebirths view birth as a natural process.

Midwifery is a respectable profession, but it falls short when it cannot empower women to make birth choices that include unassisted homebirth. Midwifery also fails every time it encourages birth to be a woman's issue and excludes the husband. Alister Hunt, along with many others, believes that childbirth is no time to leave the husband on the sideline; he needs to be an active participant.

"When interviewing prospective midwives," says Alister,

> we realized that childbirth is viewed [by midwives] as an experience that women share, rather than an experience that a husband and wife share. It constantly surprised us that women assumed that the shared experience of childbirth was a bond that surpassed the marital bond. The surprisingly high tear rate reported by midwives indicated to me that midwife-assisted delivery lacked something in patience and/or relaxation.

David Stewart, author of *The Five Standards of Safe Childbearing* supports midwifery.

> The idea of a midwife as a knowledgeable, helpful, sympathetic skilled supporter and helper of the laboring mother has been tested throughout the ages and is of proven good. The idea of doctoring as a highly trained intervener who can induce the onset of labor, speed or delay its progress, or bring about a controlled termination by surgery is a very new approach to birth, one that has not been tested and which has not yet been proven good as a general approach to birth. (Stewart 1997: 73)

Gwen Rankin, former chairman of the National Childbirth Trust offers an opinion that many agree with:

> I would say that a fair proportion of our midwives in their thirties and forties are really frustrated doctors at heart, women very keen about taking control of labor and extremely enthusiastic about obstetric techniques. They are superb deliverers of babies, wonderful at giving injections,

and they approach birth as obstetricians do. (Arms 1975: 261)

Overall, most midwives want to see women having safe, satisfying childbirth experiences. There are more midwives than doctors who are willing to offer prenatal services to couples who opt for a DIY homebirth. However, do not expect support from a midwife when you have chosen to birth alone.

A supporter, a friend

Midwives get to know the couple more intimately and appear more compassionate than traditional obstetricians. It is much more common for the pregnant woman to become friends with her midwife than with her doctor. Midwives sometimes offer free services and information to pregnant women. They are in business to make money, but tend to value helping others. You are more likely to encounter a midwife rather than a doctor who will negotiate a fee for services.

A new mother will treasure the midwife who has been truly caring and respectful of the family unit, perhaps because the midwife is a woman or spends more time than a doctor with the expectant mother. Still, it depends on the personalities involved. The midwife decides whether to allow friendships to form with clients. Some midwives discourage emotional attachments, forming instead, a cordial, business relationship with their clients.

Like obstetrics, childbirth is a business for midwives. A sense of loss (of friendship) accompanies every birth, especially for women who formed a special bond with their midwife during the prenatal period. The midwife friend who spent a lot of time during the last few months will need to spend time with new clients.

Mistakes are possible in any human endeavor. There are various levels of competence in all fields of work. Values and ego needs will affect how she approaches her job as a midwife. A midwife with strong ego needs may want to control the birth event and could feel threatened or insulted that a couple would plan a DIY homebirth. At best, midwives can be a great source of strength and support for the laboring woman in addition to providing medical expertise.

Holistic approach

I would rather see more women seeking the services of midwives than obstetricians. There was a time when I viewed doctors as professional experts who had a higher educational background, more training, and a higher degree of expertise than midwives. Midwives are better suited for normal pregnancies and births while OB/Gyns are skilled at handling difficult cases. However, neither profession should be idolized and one is not necessarily better than the other. The individual practitioner should be interviewed by the expectant couple to determine compatibility.

We need to scrutinize how the doctor's training and experience contributes to his philosophy and actual practice of delivering babies. What exactly is his educational background preparing him for? His approach to prenatal care and beliefs about childbirth indicate how labor and delivery will transpire.

Doctors are taught to treat illness and pain. Focus is on scientific, medical procedures. Midwives are also concerned with scientific, medical procedures, but encompass a holistic approach. They are generally concerned with overall health, both physically and psychologically. Midwifery is prevention-oriented rather than treatment-oriented.

Obstetrics relies on women's low self-esteem, passivity, and ignorance of fertility and the birth process. Because of this, women perceive themselves as being unhealthy and uninformed, in need of obstetrics. Since the myths of childbirth are believed by a large number of people, thousands of women may not consider unassisted homebirth as a viable alternative.

Midwifery encourages confidence and education. While OB/Gyns prescribe artificial contraception and use drugs during childbirth, midwives encourage women to understand their fertility cycles and to cope with labor and delivery in a natural setting. Non-pharmacological methods of pain relief and herbal remedies are her tools.

Proactive prenatal care

Most women choose an OB/Gyn upon discovering a pregnancy. They will subject themselves and their unborn child to a series of prenatal appointments. During these appointments they may wait a long period of time and be subjected to tests which are sometimes inaccurate and risky. Tests have their place in prenatal care, but not at the expense of causing women and their unborn child stress, anxiety or harm. Good prenatal care is important, but for a woman who has an extremely healthy pregnancy, ten to fifteen visits to the OB/Gyn does not reap many benefits.

Questions a midwife asks during a prenatal appointment include: "How is your nutrition? Are you getting enough exercise and rest? How are you feeling emotionally? Are you doing your Kegel exercises and perineal massage?" A doctor's chart records nausea, swelling and headaches. There's no need to take a proactive approach when there are treatments that will solve various problems (which may not have been problems in the first place if a proactive approach was taken). Business practices by doctors involve processing patients quickly. Pregnant women often look forward to the outside educational classes, where they get more attention and reassurance.

Midwives often travel to the couple's home to conduct prenatal visits. A couple planning a DIY homebirth may form a personal relationship or sign a contract for limited services with a midwife. These services might include initial blood work, one or two prenatal appointments and agreement that the midwife will serve as a back-up if the couple decides against an unassisted homebirth.

The prenatal process can be personal, informative and special with a midwife. An expectant couple blossoms emotionally because the pregnant woman feels she is cared for much more deeply by the midwife than a doctor. The devoted midwife feels privileged to know the expectant mother. Because some midwives approach birth as just a job where the couple is privileged to employ her, the couple's interviewing process must be structured so as to rule out this type of midwife.

Educational advisor

Many couples planning unassisted homebirths do not seek prenatal care from anyone. A midwife is often an excellent resource because of her network with others devoted to childbirth. She can introduce labor coaches, doulas, childbirth educators or women with similar problems to a couple planning a DIY birth.

Midwives can provide a strong bond among women in the months leading up to childbirth. We desperately need to strengthen our knowledge, pass it around more freely and ensure that we do not eliminate the essence of childbirth. So much is given over to the experts in hopes that they will take care of us, that those who are educated must make an effort to help others, especially the next generation.

Midwives are in a position to reverse the trend of childbirth ignorance in our culture. Doctors represent one level of expertise, and midwives represent another. Midwifery information emphasizes natural birth at home while obstetrics focuses on drugs and hospital birth. The ultimate goal should be for women to share information with women and for spouses to share their pregnancy and birth together. In essence, we could all be moving towards eliminating obstetrics and midwifery—not a popular goal for the baby professionals, but immensely beneficial to couples.

As women have more babies, they tend to trust their bodies' ability to function throughout pregnancy and feel no need for traditional prenatal care. They develop their own prenatal program or seek advice from a network of friends. Whatever the situation, we should all respect a couple's intelligence, experience, and right to choose. Homebirthers are not only filled with love, wisdom and common sense, but they take birth very seriously. They make a major clearly understood commitment, not just a whimsical decision to have a baby at home.

An unassisted birth requires research and education. The dedicated work of the midwives throughout the years has provided couples with a plethora of information. There are several books, magazines, newsletters and other resources written by midwives that can help any couple with all of their concerns. Midwives who attend homebirths have a wealth of experience that can be passed on to other men and women.

The contributions from people such as social anthropologist Sheila Kitzinger and obstetrician Michel Odent have been unparalleled. Ina May Gaskin and many others have had phenomenal success in midwifery in the United States. Their publications and ideas would greatly benefit anyone deciding to have an attended or unattended homebirth.

Why midwives oppose unassisted homebirth

A couple who has decided to have a DIY homebirth has basically admitted that they do not want or feel they need a midwife at their birth. Many midwives do not support unassisted births and will not agree to help a woman throughout the pregnancy, during a birth emergency, or for a postpartum examination. Some midwives feel that the couple is taking a moderate or high risk by not having medical attention during childbirth, while others feel that a DIY is a professional insult to them and their many years of training.

A segment of the midwifery profession may feel that unassisted homebirth is fine for some people, but they believe that the vast majority of women should seek medical attention for an event as crucial as childbirth. The general public, they assume, is just not smart or skilled enough to take matters into their own hands. Hence, the need for midwives.

Midwives who perpetuate the myth that childbirth is inherently dangerous are acting irresponsibly. It is detrimental to prospective parents when either midwives or obstetricians say that women need their services. Unfortunately, the public is apt to believe the professionals.

Midwives oppose unassisted births when the pregnancy is high-risk. Perhaps the woman is extremely overweight with gestational diabetes and has had several problems with previous pregnancies and deliveries. Because perceptions and opinions vary, there will always be disagreement about what constitutes a safe birth and what is high-risk.

Many DIYers are overly cautious about healthy pregnancies and safe deliveries. Those who would never entertain the idea of a DIY birth are not so much cautious as they are uninformed, fearful or conformant. Doctors and midwives often perpetuate the myth that DIYers are callous, irresponsible and act in unsafe manners.

It is not uncommon for midwives to attribute "luck" to a successful DIY, while calling attention to an unusual DIY with problematic outcomes. When a midwife I spoke with discovered that I had an unassisted homebirth, she portrayed my successful DIY as an exception rather than the rule. "So much can go wrong with the cord or the placenta. Women need a loving, caring, educated facilitator. There's a lot more to birth than reading a few books, taking some classes and using positive mind control. I know a couple who's baby was born with irreversible brain damage." I pointed out that babies are born with all kinds of problems in spite of place, technology or attendant. An unassisted homebirth does not carry added risks that would result in a disabled child.

I also found it very interesting that she admitted that a few of her own children were DIY births. I don't know whether to consider that as hypocrisy, arrogance, or competence. I imagine that midwives who have experienced beautiful DIY births would not care to share this joy with other women, potential clients.

Midwives whose priority is making money will harbor resentment towards the DIY community and view the growing population of DIYers as taking business from them. Midwives who value money over all else will eventually compete with other midwives for customers, reducing midwifery to a system not unlike "assembly-line obstetrics." The unfortunate result would be less service to women and the loss of special relationships midwives often form with clients. This would result in a breakdown in childbirth options, creating a void. Someone who is too competitive rather than sincerely helpful is probably not someone you want at your birth.

Laura Kaplan Shanley recalls a speaking engagement.

> A midwife had asked me to come to a gathering she was having of current and prospective clients. She agreed with much of my philosophy concerning unassisted birth and felt these women would be interested. When I got there I began speaking to them about some of my beliefs. After a few minutes, the midwife's partner called me into the other room and told me that although she agreed with much of what I was saying, she wanted me to only speak when spoken to, and only to that individual woman. Two of the women in the group had yet to decide whether to go with these midwives. These women were more conventional and the midwife was afraid they would be frightened by my ideas. There was also a woman there who had read my book and was thinking about having an unassisted birth. Basically, the midwife told me, she was afraid I was costing her business.

Why midwives are unnecessary

Recognizing that midwives serve a valuable purpose, DIYers still decide to not employ them. Why? The answer to this question depends on what the couple's goal is for their childbirth experience and what their philosophies are about pregnancy and childbearing.

In order to understand why a midwife is unnecessary, let us review what an unassisted birth is in a psychological context. A birth event where only the couple is present is the ultimate in intimacy and freedom.

A couple who conceives a child in a private, intimate manner and then bears a child in a private intimate manner achieves what very few other couples experience. They often achieve what psychologist Abraham Maslow has described as self-actualization. Many couples cannot conceive of a more intense peak experience equal to or greater than a DIY homebirth. After our DIY homebirth, my husband felt that his life was complete and conceded that there was probably nothing left in life to come close to our birth experience.

A couple who births a child in the same privacy in which they conceived the child strengthens their union and is more likely to achieve sexual fulfillment. Making love should be a private, personal affair and the ultimate result of that joining together, birthing a baby, should be done in a modest setting. It is the most healthy scenario in achieving femininity and masculinity. The presence of a midwife inhibits this achievement and detracts from the true experience of childbirth at its core element. Childbirth is and should be approached as a sexual experience. Since I would not want a midwife present while making love with my husband, I do not want a midwife present while having a baby with my husband.

Those who are mentally and physically confident in their ability to give birth will not feel a need to employ medical practitioners. Those who desire a DIY will need to develop the strength to avoid anyone who questions or seeks to destroy confidence. At the same time, they must maintain a healthy pregnancy or admit the need for a skilled attendant. Unassisted birth is possible for everyone, but very difficult for some.

Couples who thought they needed a midwife have sometimes admitted after their baby's birth that she was not necessary. The couple could have had a DIY birth. Midwives may be able to offer assistance, but are bound by limitations. In the event of a complication, such as a prolapsed cord, a midwife has to transport the mother to the hospital.

> A midwife's potential usefulness does not outweigh the possible disruptive factor—even if she's quiet as a mouse in the next room. You certainly won't *forget* she's there.
> —Cindy Earley-Steinke

Women need love and kindness for their birth experience and the best place to find that is with their lovers, not some midwife or doctor. If more people considered love and kindness as a prerequisite for their births, they would realize that they do not need to invite anyone to their homes who may impose rules and regulations.

Sex, love and birth are for lovers. We have too many forces in our society working against the sanctity, modesty and intimacy of couples. Don't be fooled by those midwives who have an agenda of their own.

When a midwife is needed

A midwife is needed as long as the couple perceives that she is needed. Couples who feel comfortable with their midwife and fully trust her will feel a high degree of fulfillment at their birth. Because some pregnancies and deliveries will be more risky than others and medical attention may be needed, many people faced with an upcoming birth will not feel secure doing it on their own. Different people have varying comfort levels. I would discourage couples from having a DIY if they felt unsafe or frightened without a midwife present. A child who fears the dark should not be forced to sleep in the dark, but be given a night light.

In support of my midwife

Wendy and Matt Bunkelman had the utmost respect for their midwife even though she arrived a few minutes after the birth of Abigail. They had a detailed contract, clear verbal communication, and a pleasant friendship. Wendy's midwife provided excellent prenatal care and stayed with the Bunkelman's for eight hours after the birth. She assisted with the placenta, conducted a newborn exam, cleaned up and helped celebrate. She visited the next day, three days later and when the baby was a week old. The midwife gave her a postpartum exam at six weeks. Although they managed just fine without their midwife, the Bunkelman's will probably use a midwife at their next birth.

My unprofessional midwife

Kim and Frank Pratt called their midwife when Kim was in labor and the midwife said, "I promise I'll be there." Unfortunately the midwife did not make it. Soon after the baby was born, the apprentice arrived. She was young, childless and had not been to many births, so she waited until the midwife arrived. The midwife arrived, made demands and insisted that Frank put on gloves to handle his baby.

She didn't stay very long and never apologized. She asked for the final payment when the Pratt's attended her engagement party the next month. Frank felt angry and Kim was disappointed that the midwife befriended her throughout the pregnancy and turned cold after the birth.

Several months later, Kim discovered that the midwife was arrested because she was at a birth, illegally, and the baby was stillborn. The midwife had been making comments about not trusting pregnant women and that she was tired of being on call all of the time.

Hiring a midwife

When a couple decides to employ a midwife, they are making a hiring decision. A couple should not place themselves in a subservient role to the midwife, whether it is before or after finalizing a service agreement.

During the selection process, the couple has complete control in decision-making. Once a midwife has been chosen, she will be paid for her contribution towards the birth. Although the couple has some say in their birth, they are bound by regulations and priorities set by the midwife.

Finding a midwife

Finding a midwife to attend a homebirth may pose difficulties for women. It is highly unlikely that traditional medical sources will reveal or even know about midwives in the community. Many midwives do not advertise in the yellow pages or anywhere, preferring to operate by word-of-mouth and keeping a low profile.

You may find a midwife through a local, national or international organization. Many childbirth educators and La Leche League organizations in your local community may know of midwives who attend homebirths. Other possible sources: chiropractor, homeschool organization, homeopathic practitioner, health food store, Christian or alternative bookstore.

You may find resources in unusual places and through people you would not normally imagine. I can recall at least three instances in my life of finding important information through people I did not think very highly of or did not expect would be able to help. It is very important to be a good listener; do not underestimate the value of small talk. Even that inconsiderate, irritable neighbor who plays loud music may provide you with the name of an important contact.

Ask specific questions. Many decide upon a midwife after they have "heard" that she has a good reputation. Find out why someone thinks a particular person has a good reputation. You might get more information if you stated, "I'm looking for a midwife who will not make me submit to four blood tests, who will be very quiet at my birth and who understands that I like to dance around the house naked while I'm in labor. Do you know of anyone who might fit my needs?" Know what you want in a midwife before you begin your search. Without clear goals, you will be swept away in the excitement and your goals may end up not being your own, but those of the midwife.

Some questions to ask

You will undoubtedly have several questions to ask a midwife during your first meeting. Here are a few more to add to your list:

History. Why are you a midwife? How and why did you get

started? Why are you doing it now? Do you have kids and what were their birth circumstances (C-section, another midwife at home, unassisted, etc.)? How many years have you been a midwife?

Current practice. How many births per month do you attend? What do you do when you arrive? What do you expect from couples? How do you include the father in the birth? Tell me about some of your failures and successes. Give me the names of two or three people who were unhappy with your services and two or three people who were satisfied with your services. Do you have a videotape of a birth you attended? Have you ever missed a birth and how did you handle it? Have you ever been sued or taken to court? Have you taken any clients to court and why? Have you ever terminated a relationship with a client and why?

Try to find out why someone might have fired the midwife. Determine if she networks at the local and state level. There may be a good reason why childbirth educators do not mention the name of the only midwife in town.

Your job is that of a detective. You are trying to uncover as much as you can so that you can make smart decisions now and avoid problems later.

Personality and character

Hiring mistakes occur when you consider competence without placing any value on dependability, honesty and commitment. You can assess these qualities during your initial interview, as well as by asking others who have witnessed her at a birth.

Determine what the midwife will "allow." She may require that you go to a hospital of her choice if labor is progressing slowly. If you want a doctor to provide back-up medical expertise in case of an emergency and the midwife will not agree to that, you should not compromise what you feel will be in your best interests. Undue stress and anxiety are to be avoided during the pregnancy.

Was the midwife on time for her initial meeting with you? Was she willing to share information? Did she present herself in a positive and professional manner? Did she seem realistic and honest?

If you are hoping for a wonderful birth at home and overlook a midwife who is tardy, exaggerates, or is aggressive during your initial or prenatal appointments, you will probably feel disappointed. You will still be "hoping" for that perfect birth experience. Pay attention to even the most minor nuances to prevent against nuisances. Do not disregard your intuitive feelings about the midwife.

Signing a contract

Signing a contract should not be viewed as the beginning of a business relationship, but should mark the end of a thorough search. Hopefully, a reciprocal friendship can emerge during the course of forty weeks. It might even benefit couples to meet with midwives *before* a desired pregnancy. If you treat birth as an intimate event, you should share it only with those you are very close with. Continuing a relationship with a midwife after the birth might make you decide to employ her services at your next birth.

Both parties should be cautious when agreeing on payment. Some midwives are not paid when couples transport to the hospital or are very dissatisfied about the birth. Many midwives expect full payment before the birth, and, when they do not show up for the birth, they will not reimburse the couple. If that is what was agreed upon in the contract, the couple should comply and not complain. The negotiating should take place before signing a contract.

A contract represents expectations. Expectations should be clearly communicated and everyone involved should be professional enough to honor those expectations. Midwives will soon become discouraged at serving a financially derelict community. Midwives who are derelict in their duties will develop an unfavorable reputation. Litigation or small claims court is not the answer and everyone loses when promises are not kept.

Couples need to plan for a midwife's absence at their birth. You can bet that midwives have a strategy for dealing with clients who do not pay. What about the midwife who fails to show up at a birth? I have known a few couples who have had unplanned, unattended homebirths and others who went to the hospital. In some cases the midwives promised to be there. Some midwives falsely assumed that labor would progress slowly because it was inconvenient for them to get to the couple's home quickly. Other midwives later stated that, "It was God's will that I did not make it." They never conceded that it was "God's will" to apologize, take responsibility for their failure to show, or pay back a portion of the fee.

Midwives can be expectant parents' special friends. We must not forget their contribution to society. Midwives act as educators, advisors, friends, supporters, and experts. Without these individuals to serve pregnant women, many "secrets" would not be passed down through the generations.

When it comes to birthing, couples need a suitable environment, that's all. My message is, "Kibitzers, keep out!"
—Marilyn Moran

16

Childbirth: A Feminist Issue?

Female sexuality is about love and birth and creating life....
It is an expression of the greatest female power. (Mann
1994: 240)

The most significant event in a woman's life—childbirth—has been largely ignored by the feminists. Well
known feminists are silent about this event, which will be
experienced by a majority of women at some point in their
lives. Are they aware of the maltreatment of women during
pregnancy and childbirth? If their silence is deliberate, it
would be fair to label their lack of concern as insensitive. We
could then be justified in accusing feminists of a selfish
agenda—one that does not include birth.

My search for feminist writings revealed very little interest or discussion about birth. Pregnancy is usually discussed
in the context of avoidance or problems. Teen pregnancies,
abortion and battered pregnant women emerge as passionate topics. Artificial contraception was more likely to be
discussed rather than fertility awareness or how women can
have empowered births. Feminists are more reactive than
proactive, reacting to the perceived threat of a woman's rights
being taken away, rather than seeking a woman's right to fulfillment.

268 Unassisted Homebirth

Brackhill, Rothman and Armstrong, as well as many other birth advocates encourage women to avoid the exploitations of traditional childbirth. Just because the leaders of the feminist movement do not talk about dignified and empowered birth does not mean we should disregard the issue.

Who are the feminists and what do they advocate?

The term "feminism" is practically synonymous with radicalism; many women are reluctant to identify with it. Women reap the benefits, yet distance themselves from the feminist movement, which has been partially responsible for improvements during the past forty years. We cannot deny the fact that women have profited from participation in the workforce, better pay, and more independence and self-confidence in their lives than ever before. Equal opportunity, less discrimination and enforcement of sexual harassment violations are also the result of hard work by dedicated feminists.

With freedom comes responsibility to make intelligent choices. Freedom backfires if choices are made in the absence of morality, concern for others, or concern for consequences. We are free to murder and steal, but they are not sensible actions. Some individuals feel threatened as others gain power. They are so preoccupied with their own insecurities that they fail to realize that increased freedoms can coexist for all. As freedom increases for one, it does not necessarily decrease for another.

Feminists seek to secure rights and opportunities available to men, with reproductive and employment issues being key priorities. Feminists value independence and choices which will benefit their lives or their families and they are willing to challenge the system as they fight for principles that will improve women's lives.

Sherrye Henry, author of *Deep Divide: Why American Women Resist Equality,* found that although many women define themselves as nonfeminists, equality issues are important to them. Many of these women perceive feminism as an anti-male, anti-child movement. In her efforts to educate the public about what feminism includes, Henry says there are at least three distinct feminist philosophies: radical feminism, social feminism and women's rights feminism.

Radical feminism blames men for female inequality. Women who feel oppressed and excluded may feel angry and resentful.

The biologically determined roles of bearing children and nursing them are perceived as negative, unless the pregnancy is planned and desired. Radicals believe that women remain dependent upon men in traditional family structures and view this as a major deterrent to women's economic and overall power. Thus, any options which free women of their dependent status are desirable. Birth control, test-tube insemination and fertilization techniques are reproductive options that free women from men. Radical feminists believe that the oppression of women is fostered by marriage and motherhood.

While radicals see men as oppressors, social feminists view the economic class system as the problem. Social feminists equate a woman's worth with the amount of her paycheck. Family responsibilities are augmented—and in some cases replaced—by child care and other social institutions. Radical and social feminists prefer to ignore childbirth and motherhood altogether.

Women's rights feminism has no programmed ideology like the other two, but rests on the principle that all people are created equal and deserve equal opportunity. Women's rights feminism is not embraced by everyone; some feel that women do not need any additional rights. They believe there is nothing wrong that must be corrected.

Political and economic clout are main goals of feminism, but so is an insistence on bringing dignity and respect to women. Christina Hoff Sommers asserts that only one out of four women defines herself as a feminist. She attributes the problem of modern day feminism, or "Second Wave Feminism," to being too radical. She accuses leaders of the feminist movement of preaching that women are trapped in male dominance, or "heteropatriarchy." These "gender feminists" believe that institutions (whether it be the state, family or schools) perpetuate male dominance.

Sommers believes that over ninety percent of today's women support "First Wave" feminism, built on the foundations of equity and fair treatment without discrimination. Unfortunately, most people think of feminism today as Second Wave.

Whether a woman describes herself as a feminist or traditionalist is insignificant when you consider the basic human rights that unite us all. A family-centered traditional woman and a career-centered Second Wave Feminist would both agree that women have the right to birth and mother their children in their own way. All women have a strong desire to be recognized as an important part of society, not to be taken for granted or abused.

"The Second Stage"

> The second stage cannot be seen in terms of women alone, our separate personhood or equality with men. The second stage involves coming to new terms with the family—new terms with love and with work. The second stage may not even be a women's movement. Men may be at the cutting edge of the second stage. The second stage has to transcend the battle for equal power in institutions. The second stage will restructure institutions and transform the nature of power itself. The second stage may even now be evolving, out of or even aside from what we have thought of as our battle. (Friedan 1981: 28)

In *The Second Stage*, Betty Friedan admits that the feminists need to change direction in order to make progress. She believes that she lived through an era when the feminist cycle was broken and that "it won't be finished until our daugh-

---

Feminists believe that reproductive freedom has everything to do with not having a baby and nothing to do with actually having one! —Laura Kaplan Shanley

ters can freely, joyously choose to have children." (Friedan 1981: 36). She acknowledges that being a mother brings about "uneasiness, unsureness and fear."

While we can exert control in many facets of our lives, there are a few of which we are not fully in control. Child-bearing and many facets of childrearing are among those few. We are venturing on uncharted waters in our lives each time we give birth and as our children mature.

Winning an undeclared war and competing (especially with men) to achieve a certain level of power are goals of the feminists. When we compete, we all, men or women, use our special talents and skills to be better than someone else. We also try to become like others in order to compete on their playing field. Competition and selfishness do not contrib-ute to unity with spouses, families and communities. If we try to become like men, the qualities of womanhood will get in our way. In a sense, feminism is a denial or repression of womanhood.

We need to praise womanhood and coexist as separate and unequal. Until we admit that women are superior to and unique from men regarding many physical capabilities, we will not be able to celebrate womanhood. Likewise, men are superior to women in many physical ways. We have to stop competing and lowering our respect by trying to erase dif-ferences.

Mothers who embrace their roles are not trapped. Those who stay home and raise their children have chosen to take full responsibility for our next generation.

Women who feel it is their duty and obligation to become a mother have not established an identity outside a perceived role. The same would be true of an unhappy career-focused woman. Spending over forty hours a week in any job where you do not have the freedom to be yourself can be viewed as

---

I think we must at least begin to openly discuss feminist denial of the importance of family, of women's own needs to give and get love and nurture, tender loving care. —Betty Friedan

a trap. We are trapped if we are not allowed to exercise our free will.

Friedan reminds us that the feminists of the 1920's were either single or career women and did not have to reconcile demands of family and career. They were against motherhood, marriage, family, sexual intimacy with men and any traits or behaviors which pleased and attracted men.

Today, the feminist goal is self-realization in whatever a woman chooses to do. However, Friedan accuses women of not taking risks. We prefer to exert control and keep our vulnerabilities hidden. It seems less risky to pursue a career than to take on a major life responsibility of bearing and raising children. Thus, birth and mother issues are not important.

Why childbirth has been ignored by the feminists

Sherrye Henry discovered that many feminists are disenchanted with the way the movement presents itself. One-third of self-described feminists were either uninvolved or alienated,

> perhaps because a large majority of feminists agree with mainstream women about the best part of being female: 63 percent of the feminists and 65 percent of mainstream women answered 'being a mother.' Clearly, the feminist leadership has a job to do, both with its own followers and with all the newcomers who are just ripe for the picking. (Henry 1984: 271)

Henry's research revealed what most of us already know: motherhood is a prominent part of a woman's life. Radical and social feminists devalue motherhood and in doing so, they neglect birth. A new self emerges with the birth of a child and the feminists couldn't care less.

Childrearing detracts from the amount of time available to dedicate to a career. Women, the minority, need money to gain power so that they position themselves with men, the majority. Since natural mothering is not a paid profession, motherhood is of little value to the feminists. Full time mothers sense that they are useless to feminist causes and often do not identify with feminism.

The more prominent one's professional title, the greater likelihood of wielding power. Women who devote energy to their professions have spent a lot of time preparing, training and educating themselves. The dedication it takes to be a professional working woman does not leave much time for motherhood. It is a rare woman who can excel at all roles, simultaneously. A superior support system must be in place along with an ability to balance priorities.

We must decide whether we are going to balance family, career and personal pursuits simultaneously or if we will focus on one component at a time. Feminists often chose careers over motherhood. Birth and "homeworking" alone are not championed; but issues combining motherhood and careers are. Day care, family leave, maternity leave, and sick time to care for a child or parent are primary concerns.

Those who are consumed by motherhood often do not have time to commit to feminist issues, while the vocal feminists who do have time uphold non-birth issues. Some people portray feminists as abortion rights advocates trying to be like men, but feminists are not just bitter, angry women clawing their way to break through the glass ceiling in male-dominated professions. They have families and are employed in various vocations. Most feminists do not resent men, but are simply dissatisfied with the prevalent power inequities.

The right to choose

> For many years women in the US have been concentrating their efforts on informing both men and women about women's reproductive rights. However, in their fight for their reproductive rights, women have left an important and basic issue by the wayside: freedom of choice during pregnancy and childbirth; the right to have a nonmedicalized labor and delivery, free from unnecessary intervention and technology. Giving birth is a function that women inherently know how to perform, if left alone for nature to take

its course. Women also need to take responsibility for themselves and to not be afraid of their bodies. Their bodies were made to give birth for the continuation of the species. There is no mystery about it. If women educate themselves about birth and trust in their bodies, they will suffer fewer complications for both themselves and their babies. (Napierala 1994: 6)

The right to choose abortion allows us to decide whether a particular life is of value. Courageous women have fought for the right to choose pregnancy and abortion. Now we need to encourage women to take a stand during prenatal care and childbirth. For those who choose to give birth in a hospital, that means, asserting your rights as a patient. It means being knowledgeable and educated about childbirth. It means not letting others make decisions for you. It means not submitting to tests, technology and medication without thoroughly understanding the risks and the effects to you and your baby.

A prenatal test that reveals an abnormality incurs anxiety and requires a decision to continue or terminate the pregnancy. There may be subtle pressure from medical personnel to choose what they deem as socially appropriate. That often means destroying a fetus, which no one will ever know for sure was abnormal. As we seek to manipulate situations, we do not want imperfections. When abnormalities occur, we do not accept them very well.

Emphasis on abortion

Feminists have not fully challenged the patriarchal and totalitarian medical system. They have mainly criticized the male-dominated workplace and family structure. A patriarchal family structure is oppressive for women who believe that work in the home is menial. Some believe that women must wield as much power as men. The way to achieve this is for women to have full control over their lives and their bodies. That is why the abortion issue is the main focus of the feminists even more so than equal pay for one's work.

If abortion were illegal, women would not have the right to terminate a pregnancy, i.e., control their own bodies. Birth is not as important to the feminists because women are not denied anything tangible during the birth process. Feminists are concerned that women have the choice to give birth, not whether the birth process is rewarding and non-exploitative.

Just the fact that our society accepts abortion indicates that we are living in an anti-child, anti-mother society. The act of abortion is selfish because the desires and needs of the self are put above all others. Of course, abortion rights advocates argue that in many cases, a child will devastate—usually economically—an unmarried teenager's life or poor woman's life; therefore, many women are better off aborting their unborn. After all, feminists believe that economic power is the means to a greater power.

Abortion is anti-woman since it often harms women psychologically and sometimes medically. Abortion gives men license to behave irresponsibly and take women for granted sexually. A resulting pregnancy does not really matter since abortion is a simple way to solve the problem. Women are more likely than men to grieve or experience post-abortion syndrome. Men are left powerless when their partners decide to abort without their consent. Abortion is often the only issue which keeps anti-abortionists from identifying with feminism.

Social conditioning

Young girls are taught many social behaviors which are carried into adulthood. Cliques and conformist behaviors are rewarded. Originality and deviation from the norm can result in a girl's being ousted from the group and left feeling lonely. Ideas that are original and contributions that can make a monumental difference will not be respected since they cannot find a place within the status quo. Excelling is not an enviable goal.

Women who are pregnant with their first child are often concerned with selecting baby names, maternity clothes, decorating a nursery, whether to breastfeed or bottlefeed and how to work a baby into their current lifestyle. They will most likely attend a class sponsored by the hospital where they are subtly taught how to be a good patient and how to birth their babies according to hospital policies, rather than natural tendencies.

Many women value harmony, compromise and service to others. They do not want to upset people they respect; they are also uncomfortable upsetting those they do not respect. Offending others, appearing "too" smart, and other socially unacceptable behaviors are avoided. Because of our social conditioning, we are submissive in the birth process. Many patients look to the doctor to make decisions about administering drugs, inducing labor or performing a C-section.

Social conditioning has resulted in a system where doctors are problem-solvers and the patients are recipients, causing many women not to collaborate with their doctors during their births, but rather obey instructions. Some women are fortunate to have a hospital birth that is one of mutual participation, with everyone working toward a common goal. Although many childbirth educators encourage the couple to write a birth plan, these plans are not taken seriously unless the couple is assertive. Hospitals are in business to make money, not to cater to a laboring woman's inner needs and desires.

Some have suggested that obstetrics is a field with a high number of misogynists. Patients are often condescended to, ignored, poked, prodded and treated as a machine. Women have been conditioned to exert control over pain and to suppress the expression of it.

During the delivery of my first child, the nurse told me not to panic. I was not panicking, but simply expressing pain. I wondered why an experienced OB nurse would not recognize the basic sounds of childbirth. I figured it was probably because her experience consisted of drugs used to silence the normalcy of birth. After my nonmedicated second birth, the nurse recommended that I "take something next time." In fact, her tone was so authoritarian, as if she was trying to make me promise that I would take drugs to escape from childbirth.

She probably couldn't handle my authenticity either. I later found out that she was an alcoholic. Perhaps alcohol was her way to escape from the difficulties of life. Throughout most of my births the nurses would continuously ask if I wanted drugs, expecting me to comply, before I progressed to the next stage of labor.

After four hospital deliveries, I was conditioned to rely on internal vaginal exams as a primary indication of labor progression. I thought that the doctor needed to first determine and then tell me when it was appropriate to push. While planning for our unassisted homebirth, I thought it would be crucial to check my cervix for dilation. I began to take steps to learn how to do this. Then I learned that frequent checking can actually slow the progression of labor and cause an infection. During a few of my births, it was very painful for a doctor the check my body's readiness. I had one doctor who was about 6'4," with large hands. I was in such physical pain that I yanked his hand out of me. I got a polite scolding from the nurse who mentioned restraining me or tying me down if I continued interfering with the doctor's ability to do his job.

"Why do we need to check the readiness for pushing?" is what I asked myself while preparing for our last birth. Should we force ourselves against nature or let the baby do most of the work? I did not have to push very much during my first four births and decided that I would let the baby do most of the work on its own. I would not push until I had an uncontrollable urge.

Women feel uncomfortable and ambivalent about claiming power in their relationships with their doctors. Those who question the status quo or make extraordinary demands will encounter resistance. I might have been viewed as an uninformed, threatening or rebellious patient throughout the years. The questions I asked were too confrontational or trite for the workers. With my second child, I asked a nurse if the result of the AFP test was used as a tool to make an abortion decision and she said, "No. A medevac helicopter will be ready to transport the newborn to a specialized hospital." I declined the test because of its high inaccuracy rate and figured that medevac helicopters are on standby regardless of any test result. One doctor admitted to me that in his twenty-five years of practice, the only problem he had was the high amount of false positive results. The AFP test indicated a deformity, but all of his patients delivered normal babies.

With other pregnancies I declined an ultrasound and showed up for less than the recommended appointments. I usually asked the question, "Is this absolutely medically necessary?" and would be asked to sign my initials when I refused various tests. Doctors made it clear that they offered all of these tests and wanted me, the patient, to not come back and blame them for a "problem" (i.e., imperfect baby).

It was not until I read Marilyn Moran's books, *Birth and the Dialogue of Love* (1981) and *Pleasurable Husband / Wife Childbirth: The Real Consummation of Married Love* (1997) that I knew my social conditioning needed undoing. A break with conformity and social conditioning is necessary for those who desire alternative birth.

Inequity

When we contract services with an obstetrician or midwife, we put ourselves in a subservient role. The expert has the ultimate power in childbirth since he or she will be the one to make all major decisions in an emergency. Birth is based on someone else's philosophies and goals. A woman who has hired a doctor must remember that physicians control labor and conduct delivery. The burden is on the patient to assert her desires.

Pregnant women are not always treated with respect, but are seen as a means to a financial end. But then they are not always treated with disrespect, either, but are simply customers. Insurance companies take precedence over the patient. It is easy to become complacent when others pay for our medical care. We are not held responsible and do not feel a need to question the experts and their methods. It might be a different story if we were paying our own way or asserted ourselves more easily.

There are many ways obstetricians can make more money if that is their goal. Performing more surgeries and C-sections, selling contraceptive devices, ordering tests or prescribing drugs from a company they have stock in are just a few. Any situation which can be capitalized on is fair game.

Midwives do a better job than obstetricians at forming more intimate partnerships with women, but it is ultimately a job for them too, rather than an act of kindness performed freely and generously. We are deluding ourselves if we expect more than a performance of services from doctors and midwives. We cannot pay someone and hope to have an equal partnership.

Since we do not have the ultimate power in these birth situations, we do not have full participation in our experiences and outcomes. We are often left feeling dissatisfied, incomplete and regretful. The many women who leave the hospital after a satisfying birth experience will later wonder why they cannot identify the source of their discontent or why they are suffering from postpartum depression. The reason for this is that they had established what they thought was an equal partnership with their doctor. They were mistaken. The pregnancy has come to an end and they cling to the belief that there was an equal partnership, rather than a business relationship.

Birth is a choice. Women need to know about all of their options. They need less harassment and judgment from others. Until childbirth is acknowledged as an issue worthy of attention and until women demand more from their caregivers, inequities will exist.

Faith in experts

Women have been asserting themselves for several decades in their careers and relationships. Yet, when it comes to childbirth, we are not as assertive as we could be. We want to trust the experts; it takes a burden off of us. Many people do not want to become experts because they do not have the time or desire. We are involved in too many activities and our responsibilities overwhelm us. Not only are we overwhelmed by the physical and emotional changes that take place during pregnancy, but we are preoccupied with finances and making room for a baby in our home and life.

As long as we continue to use their services, doctors will perceive that their expertise is wanted and needed. They encourage us to patronize their businesses. We may feel as if we benefit from their services, but the key to good health is personal knowledge and action.

A biased view of childbirth is presented to us by popular magazines, advertisers, hospitals and medical professionals. The medical profession has established itself as the legitimate authority on maternal and infant health, contraception, infertility, pregnancy, childbirth practices, postpartum management, infant feeding and childrearing. The public has eagerly accepted doctors as experts, without question. Unfortunately, in the process, we have not developed much confidence in our bodies. When we put all of our faith in others and disregard ourselves as experts, we are left feeling dependent, unconfident, inadequate and afraid.

Many people have a hard time making decisions in life, so they hire others because of their own laziness. Many adults look to psychologists for answers; they hire brokers to invest money for them and accountants to make sense of their finances. Instead of having faith in ourselves or putting forth extra effort, we turn to others. Sometimes those others feel a sense of bursting pride, eager to appear as experts in our doting eyes.

Many argue that we should be grateful for experts and their ability to perform difficult or life-saving functions. Yes,

---

Motherhood is bondage in a society that values selfishness. Motherhood is a joy and a privilege in a society that values love of others. If we want to improve the status and rights of women, we need to advocate birth practices where the customers and providers are at least on equal ground. Women should expect superior treatment during birth. If we could respect and celebrate our femininity, then maybe we would eventually have a society which rejoiced in women as childbearers and mothers.

we should. At one time in history, women died during child-birth. In addition to better nutrition and personal hygiene, medicine found answers and made discoveries which help women in need today. But medical discoveries need not be applied to healthy pregnant women. It is not until we learn to have faith in ourselves as experts will we set ourselves free from disappointment.

Exploitation and bondage

When it comes to service, expect the best and you may get it; demand the best and you will get it. Many women do not expect much from their birth attendants or place they will give birth. Until we set goals and become more asser-tive or even aggressive about our births, we will be open to exploitation. *Every woman who submits to the medical model of birth misses the opportunity to expand her life.*

Since childbirth is a multi-billion dollar industry, it is no surprise that money is the force behind birth practices. Many doctors, pediatricians, hospitals and citizens would like to maintain current childbirth practices, especially when hun-dreds of jobs are at stake in every community. The profitabil-ity of the maternity section in some hospitals has become very important to the bottom line. It is not uncommon to see hospital advertisements luring patients and doctors into their place of business.

Feminists are adamant that "government does not belong in the bedroom making personal family decisions." How-ever, midwife-assisted homebirth is illegal in many states and feminists do not seem to be working hard to ensure greater opportunity and choice regarding birth. The medical estab-lishment has been known to convince legislators of the "dan-ger" and "inferiority" of midwifery and homebirths. How sad it is that the powerful monopoly wants to control and preside over birth choices.

Women are induced and go on to deliver premature ba-bies who need special care. C-sections are performed more frequently than is medically necessary, and women are hooked up to monitors, given IVs, and forced to give birth in an uncomfortable position. They are given drugs to alleviate pain and to silence them. Women are not encouraged, shown or taught how to give birth successfully.

What will happen if feminists continue to ignore the issue of childbirth?

Feminists continue to disregard childbirth as a major women's issue as countless women submit to the current birth culture. Feminists have been concerned with women's rights, but if they are truly concerned with empowering women, they will realize that childbirth is an important rite of passage and that unassisted homebirth is one of the highest forms of liberation.

Anyone who exposes the comfortable status quo (and the majority's power base) is seen as a threat and must be silenced or ridiculed. The medical establishment does not want the unsuspecting public learning the truth. The majority may accuse the minority of being angry, irrational or irresponsible, as a way to discredit their point of view. What the medical profession fails to realize is that there are more couples who are choosing unassisted homebirth regardless of their bullying.

Feminists will become a more narrowly focused group if they do not expand their priorities to include issues which effect the majority of women, issues such as birth empowerment. Women are beginning to recognize the exploitation that currently abounds in traditional prenatal care and hospital deliveries. Feminists could be a pivotal force in raising awareness about birth practices in this country, if they only cared.

> The delivery table is no place for a woman to fight for her rights. But aligned with her mate, sympathetic doctors, and others of the "new breed" of mothers, she has the power to move mountains of technological equipment and procedures to preserve her absolute role as mother in the birth process, if only she knew it. —Suzanne Arms

PART V

Beyond the Birth Experience

17

Home Is Where The Hearth Is

I think the world is upside-down, and is suffering so much, because there is very little love in the homes and in family life. We have no time for our children, we have no time for each other; there is no time to enjoy each other.... Everybody today seems to be in such a terrible rush, anxious for greater developments and greater riches and so on, so that children have very little time for their parents. Parents have very little time for each other, and in the home begins the disruption of the peace of the world.... People who love each other fully and truly—they are the happiest people in the world. (Mother Teresa 1975: 11)

No place like home

Never in the history of America have there been so many people who are disgruntled with government, big business, institutions and large bureaucracies. Less than half of eligible voters cast their ballots in local and national elections. Many of those registered voters are well educated, yet we have become apathetic and do not place much confidence or trust in politicians and business leaders. The rapid growth in home-based businesses, homeschooling and home healthcare is an indication that Americans not only are heading home for happiness, but are becoming more self-sufficient.

The year 2000 elicits images of high technology and ultra-modernization. As our world gets faster and more complex, so does the typical birth experience. Women are induced to give birth quickly; they are given drugs to speed up a sluggish labor; they are given a C-section for "failure to progress." New machinery and techniques are invented and utilized by doctors to make their jobs easier. All this technology is making more and more patients feel shortchanged and exploited at birth; and causing them to question the medical way of doing things.

Because women are realizing that some things in life need to be more sacred and respected, natural health, homeopathy, and alternative approaches to medical treatments continue to gain popularity. More women are educating themselves about pregnancy, making more choices about their births, and taking some matters into their own hands. These new ideas and applications benefit individuals more than doctors. Many professional women even decide to leave their comfortable jobs and incomes to stay home with their children, and what began as a sacrifice often becomes a discovery of joy and happiness. As they spend time with their families, they find that life in the home offers tremendous possibilities to make meaningful contributions.

In the late 1950's, as feminists convinced women that life at home was unfulfilling, childbearing and childrearing, a central part of many women's lives, was suddenly unworthy. The idea that men's lives were more glamorous and women's work was meaningless began to gain momentum, and women began to value men's lives more than their own. They entered the workforce, emulated men's behavior and their manner of dress, and sought more sexual freedoms and opportunities. The birth rate eventually declined and it appeared as if the stay-at-home mom was becoming extinct, while selfish pursuits and self-discovery became more important than teamwork, service and sacrifice. Love for others was slowly being eroded by love for the self.

Luxury or drudgery?

We are now seeing how women's work in the home contributes to a family's sense of well-being. Although there is an increasing respect for the work women do inside the home, housework and being a stay-at-home mom is still viewed by the majority as repetitious and mindless. Many husbands appreciate the hard work their wives do in the home, but men who value money over family togetherness prefer that their wives work.

Some people think that there is a generation of women who are bitter and resentful about staying home and raising kids, assuming that they had no other choices. Lack of respect or praise for the hard work they did triggers resentment in some while others feel pride and accomplishment for their chosen lifestyle. Some people still view women who have children as dependent. Having become a society that values achievement and accomplishment based on financial success and what you do rather than who you are, the strength of your character and the contributions you make in affecting others' characters, namely children, is somehow ignored or considered insignificant.

There are considerable rewards for both parents to work outside the home. The economy thrives when consumers purchase goods. A two-income household has much more purchase power. Our social structure supports parents being outside the home. Most communities across the country offer full day kindergarten, preschool, and daycare. Employers offer programs geared towards a two-wage earning family. Government programs and children's summer programs are designed to accommodate busy working parents.

Many people seem to think that imagination, curiosity, and talent can't be used in the home, and some even wonder why a woman who had a prestigious career would want to stay home. What they fail to realize is that many of the skills a woman acquired in college and in the workplace are very useful in her home life.

I never felt so empowered, creative and responsible in my life until I stayed home with my children and began homeschooling them. I had enjoyed my past professions as an Army Officer and Human Resources Manager. It was rewarding to set and accomplish goals, and attaining success and coping with heartaches added depth to my life. Even with as much passion as I had for my career, it still did not provide the one reward I received after embracing a vocation in the home: love. I might have loved my jobs at one time or another, but it was never as intense or constant as one can love a spouse or child.

Although some people's identities and emotional investments are linked to their jobs, there is a greater opportunity to feel an inner peace about family than about a job. Giving birth and raising children are perhaps the most creative things we can do as people. Very few activities will make a more lasting impression on society than successfully raising children.

Making a home

Couples in love aim to make a comfortable home where they can share their love with no obligations to the outside world.

> A home is a place of peace, the shelter from every social injustice, contrast or disorder. When there is security and harmony within the home, everything is beautiful and bearable even if outside its walls there is noise and contradiction. When love between husband and wife is based on lofty sentiments, it can cope with every adventure or every drama of modern life. (Del Mazza 1984: 69)

Since most of us lead busy lives, our home is the place where we can restore our body and mind. It is in the home where we can contemplate the meaning of life. While we may

> While keeping very busy and active on the outside, he is passive and inert on the inside, because he rarely enters into his own heart. — Fulton Sheen

choose to work or volunteer for a particular organization and strive to make an enjoyable life outside the home, we will never be able to create as safe and secure a haven as our home.

The home is a place of tremendous freedom—the freedom to make mistakes and try new ideas, to experiment with singing, dancing, or any project and not be subject to criticism. It is where confidence can bloom. Some people do not take the time to make their home a place of comfort. They use it as a pit stop, choosing instead to spend more time outside the home engulfed in work, community activities and social functions.

Life in the home

Home is a place where most of us can find comfort and intimacy. In a stressful, troubling world, it is refreshing to have a retreat. Not only is it comfortable to give birth in our home, it is sensual. You begin to realize that life would be wonderful if you could do more from the home. DIYers place a priority on forming strong families; and building strong families starts in the home, leading many people decide to homeschool or operate a home-based business. The more time you spend in the home, the more you realize not only that there is so much to teach your children and so much to be learned, but also that there are many possibilities for accomplishment with a home-based lifestyle. Mary Pride, author of *The Way Home,* refers to "homeworking" as a lifestyle where mothers diligently center their life around God and their families. A homeworker is much more than a homemaker or housewife. For Pride, homeworking involves homeschooling and operating home-based businesses.

Unfortunately, many of us use our homes as a base of operation from which we conduct our busy lives. Families today hardly have time to get together for a daily meal or twenty minutes of meaningful conversation. Because we do not spend time talking together and problem-solving, we turn to other sources for information, advice and guidance, such as self-help books, therapy, or talk-radio psychologists.

Some people prefer to develop relationships with others through on-line computer services. While technology helps us access new information, it is a hindrance if it *replaces* the time we could be spending with our families.

Women do not seek information from their mothers or other women as often as they are apt to run to the doctor's office for information. The art of passing information from woman to woman around the kitchen table has become rarer than ever. Because we are not connected as women when it comes to childbirth, there are professionals willing to step in. Those in the childbirth industry provide women with all they need to know, and we are left believing the myths and conforming to a certain way of giving birth.

Imitating home

Home health care and assisted living communities recognize the sanctity and comforts of the home. Working from home is often more productive and enjoyable than working in an office at the company's location. Businesses and schools try to create a comfortable home-like atmosphere in some parts of their facilities. Trends are towards small units or teams as a way to increase productivity and learning at work and in school. Some parents believe that preschool and daycare programs not only imitate, but provide more than what is in their homes.

Innovations in education resemble what has been done in homeschool families for hundreds of years: high parental involvement, smaller class size, one on one instruction and child-directed learning. Retention and application of information is increased when students are given free time and space to explore the world according to their desires.

Birthing rooms in hospitals strive for a homelike atmosphere. Medical attendants realize that patients desire the comforts of home, because rooms are welcoming in their décor, monitors and medical equipment are hidden behind handsome looking furniture, and medical instruments are wheeled out just before the baby is born.

Similarities between homebirth and homeschool

When we embrace life in the home, we try to consider all of the things that can be done in or from the home. The enormous growth in home-based businesses and the surge in the number of homeschooling families are evidence that family togetherness is a priority to many people.

Homeschooling is an attractive vocation for mothers who previously enjoyed careers. They can be directly responsible for their children's education and development, while at the same time, their creativity, problem-solving and organizational skills are called into play as they determine what curriculum or approach is the most beneficial for their families. Although a college degree, work experience or teaching certificate are not necessary to homeschool, parents with these backgrounds enjoy the satisfaction of applying their past experiences to their current endeavor. Studies have shown that parents whose highest degree is a high school diploma are just as likely to be successful homeschoolers as those with college degrees. Adults whose eyes, ears, hearts and minds are ready for learning will gain new insights and skills that can be incorporated into their homeschool.

Education geared for the masses which occurs in institutions is called public education. Similarly, birth for the masses occurs in hospitals. Private schools can be compared to midwife-attended homebirth because the parents desire an improved method with a more personal approach.

While obstetrics is for the masses and midwifery is for the individual woman, unassisted homebirth is the only option where the husband and other children can be full participants during the birth. Unassisted homebirth is similar to homeschooling because the parents make decisions and reap the benefits and consequences. Homeschooling and homebirth are the only alternatives where parents accept full responsibility for the outcome.

Families may wish to recreate school at home where they develop a structured curriculum and a semi-rigid schedule. Other families "unschool," recognizing the child's natural tendency to seek information he finds interesting or needs to know.

Unschooling families do not follow prepared curriculums. Although unschoolers do not spend much time engrossed in structured learning, it doesn't mean that these households are chaotic or lack an educational vision. Parents who are fully immersed in their children's education (and lives) find creative ways to reach their goals. Their diligence enables them to unschool so that what appears to be "goofing off" is actually self-directed learning.

Proponents of homeschooling support the idea that education is best accomplished in a more natural learning environment rather than an institution. Unassisted homebirth, like unschooling, respects the natural unfolding of events.

Large families

By today's standards, a large family is one that has more than three children. In 1990, only 6% of families had more than four children. Some childbirth educators believe that a woman's body does not get accustomed to birth until they have had three babies. Since most of the population does not have more than three children, women may not achieve the confidence to have a homebirth. Others are not dissatisfied enough to make changes.

There are essentially two groups of people who want unassisted homebirths: those who know that they want to have an unassisted homebirth before they are pregnant or have children and those who have had previous births. In the second case, major beliefs and attitudes have evolved so that couples are willing to make bold choices in a culture where it is uncommon to have an unassisted homebirth.

As couples have more children, new responsibilities and tasks occupy their time and energy. It is no longer desirable

---

Who of us is mature enough for offspring before the offspring themselves arrive? The value of marriage is not that adults produce children but that children produce adults.
—Peter de Vries

or feasible to operate as if they were a two-child family. Successful large families usually produce individuals who learn the value of compromise, shared power and altruistic behaviors. Brotherly love is more likely to develop if the parents were selfless. Children lead parents into a new dimension of love calling forth new talents and levels of sacrifice.

Born at home; die at home

Part of the problem we have with various age groups not respecting each other is that there is very little contact outside peer groups during parts of our lifetime. We learn at an early age to seek those similar in age for our friends and acquaintances. Our society is very skilled at separating and institutionalizing life. Babies are born in hospitals; young children go to preschool; children are categorized by age at school; many elderly people live in convalescent homes; and we go to hospitals to die. Life, death and so much in between are removed from their natural settings. Young children witness people leaving home to have babies or to die. They often do not know or interact with many elderly people. Residents in convalescent homes do not regularly see young people other than employees and a few visitors.

Being born at home teaches family members the beauty and continuity of life. There is bound to be less fear and mystique about birth when families welcome a newborn immediately into their home rather than going to a hospital to give birth. Euphoria, rather than postpartum depression is often reported by couples who have had unassisted births.

A family that witnesses the death of an ailing family member in the comfort of their home does not have to deal with unpleasant attitudes from the medical staff or pressure to provide various treatments. The family has the privacy to express emotions and begin the grieving process in a more dignified manner. Those who have experienced birth or death at home have seen how the home offers a better psychological, spiritual, and sometimes physical alternative to an institution.

Homeschooling and home-based businesses offer a life-style where the family can be involved in each others' lives, learning, growing, and working together. Families that eliminate members from going to institutions for birth, death, school, or work improve unity rather than create separation.

Children who grow up in a home with parents who are intimately involved in their lives are apt to be successful citizens, employees, friends, spouses and parents. Parents that encourage independence produce children who are self-sufficient. Families who are more self-sufficient are less draining on society.

The fastest road to independence, however is traveled by the child who develops security during his dependent years—who can count on his mother's taking care of his needs.
—La Leche League

18

Advocacy

The most powerful movers of this revolution will be women themselves. How women give birth and how children are born are profoundly tied to our views of nature, science, health, medicine, freedom, and human—especially man-woman relationships. (Odent 1992: 118)

Although pregnancy and birth are part of a couple's experience, it is the woman who seeks medical services because it is her body which will be undergoing the process of pregnancy and birth. Until women demand change or choose alternatives, there will be no incentive to reform the current approach to childbirth.

Educators

Those who have had unassisted homebirths can serve as educators to a skeptical public. Whenever possible, men and women should share their birth stories with others, not being bashful or boastful, but serving as living examples that unassisted homebirth is possible and desirable.

We have to dispel the belief that only childbirth "experts" have credibility for passing on childbirth information. We can also raise awareness that all is not well with pregnancy and childbirth practices in this country; there is a better way. Fathers can have a great impact in the education arena. Men are more apt to listen and discuss a man's personal account of childbirth than seek a mentor, read childcare information or attend classes as faithfully as women seem to. The greatest source of sharing comes in the form of practical conversations with others who have had an unassisted homebirth. It is here that information not even in print can be found. We cannot underestimate the power of shared experiences.

What makes life in America so special is that we have choices. What choices for childbirth are being presented in our mainstream culture? How are couples being encouraged to give birth? Most likely, you'll see a monopoly at work as you observe hospital advertisements and review the maternity benefits covered by health insurance plans. Women believe they have many choices: which obstetrician and hospital to choose!

When we talk directly with our acquaintances, we find much more open-mindedness about alternative birth than we find among the medical community. That's why we need to take our message directly to couples. If we are not successful opening the minds of others, perhaps we can open their hearts to the joy and love that is possible.

The biggest impact we can make is to chip away at the myths of childbirth, as if we are sculpting a final piece which will show the beauty of birth rather than the outer surface. Take every opportunity you have to create public awareness. Speaking in front of large or small groups or writing articles are some ways to get valuable messages out to the public.

Our local newspaper printed a story about midwife-assisted homebirth and a local doctor was quoted as saying "childbirth is immensely dangerous." I wrote a letter to the editor stating that the United States is one of the most advanced countries in the world, yet ranks 20th in maternal and neonatal safety. This doesn't mean that childbirth is dangerous, but that the American approach to prenatal health and childbearing is substandard. 95% of today's global population was born at home, in the absence of obstetricians, technology or hospitals.

I went on to say that doctors who deal exclusively with high-risk pregnancies will eventually define all birth as unsafe, abnormal and something women should fear. This misrepresentation of birth is one of the biggest lies today. Pregnant women should be very cautious when dealing with doctors who believe that childbirth is dangerous. Their birth experience will most likely involve a procedure which relies on technology, drugs, induction and surgery to extract a baby. It is immoral for doctors to knowingly spread false information. Incompetence and exploitation are likely outcomes when doctors believe and base their practices on the myths of childbirth.

The wisdom shared with those less wise often falls on deaf ears; it is as if a different language is being spoken by the two parties. We must never give up on our quest to educate others. Conformists are apt to be misinformed (or uninformed) and passive rather than opinionated. Forgiveness and patience are often required when dealing with diverse opinions.

We have an opportunity to educate others in our daily conversations. If you raise a question that makes them think about an issue from a different angle, you will have been very effective. Oftentimes, we cannot get involved in long discussions with others, so a "shock statement" may serve a useful purpose. One woman told me it would be scary to have a baby at home without medical attention. I told her that after having four children in the hospital and then one at home it would be scary having a baby in the hospital. She could have discounted me as some eccentric fool, but if it got her thinking *why* I would make such comments, then maybe I did some good.

Mentors

Serving as mentors or examples to other parents is vital. Even medical practitioners can benefit from meeting couples

> If you want to create, you have to sacrifice superficiality, some security, and often your desire to be liked, to draw up your most intense insights, your most far-reaching visions. —Clarissa Pinkola Estes

298 Unassisted Homebirth

who have given birth without assistance. In addition to stopping the spread of childbirth myths, we need to encourage women to be courageous, to stand up to their doctors and anyone else who question the desirability of unassisted birth. Once we get couples thinking about their pregnancy and birth, we have to help them take the necessary risks.

We can share ideas and techniques in preparing for an unassisted homebirth, and we should welcome the opportunity to serve as an example to others so that they will gain the internal strength and confidence necessary for doing something that is not only countercultural, but scary. An unassisted homebirth seems frightening to most of the American population who views childbirth as a biological danger, rather than the cultural and behavioral ordeal it has become.

Men need to be encouraged to take an active part in childbirth. I am in favor of excluding other women and midwives from my birth experience and fully including my husband. Since I rely on my husband's involvement as we journey through parenthood, it is only natural to rely on him at birth. A doctor or midwife will not be sharing your life and should only be at the birth when a couple is not healthy enough or confident enough to have the baby on their own. When a husband or wife exclude each other during a major life event, something will be missing that can never be captured again.

Not only can we serve as mentors to those aspiring to have an unassisted homebirth, but to those who may not even have considered it. I am not suggesting that we act as recruiters, but that we identify possible "candidates," especially those who do not believe the myths of childbirth and have a certain amount of confidence, independence and enthusiasm.

Unassisted homebirth is often something couples "evolve" towards. Perhaps you know of a couple who had a hospital birth, followed by a midwife-attended homebirth, and although they preferred the homebirth, you detect a feeling of dissatisfaction. An unassisted homebirth may be just the type of birth they would welcome.

As the epitome of prenatal health and childbirth success, homebirthers are examples to doctors and midwives. Although I believe in humility and not boasting about experiences, unassisted homebirthers are sort of "superstars." They have gone outside the boundaries in search of a sovereign birth, often against tremendous opposition.

In a society where people are not accustomed to taking full responsibility for themselves, here is a group of people that is more likely than the general public to follow healthful prenatal habits. The father of the baby is usually more involved in the pregnancy and much more active at the birth. Excellent prenatal self-care and a rewarding childbirth experience lay the foundation for confident parenting and strong family relations. All of this is desirable for individuals.

> ...if she cannot find the culture that encourages her, then she usually decides to construct it herself. And that is good, for if she builds it, others who have been looking for a long time will mysteriously arrive one day enthusiastically proclaiming that they have been looking for this all along. (Estes 1992: 186)

Advocacy

Education, effort and intentions are important, but without action, we cannot forge ahead. Here are fifteen suggestions to help you take charge:

- Expose the birth myths to your friends.

- Ask *why. Why* do we give birth in the hospital with OB/ Gyns? *Why* do we take all these tests? *Why* do we give birth laying down? By asking provocative questions, we may help others find new solutions. More importantly, we should encourage others to think and constantly search for improved methods; but we should not tell someone how or what to think. Be a researcher. Question the experts. Rather than a doctor, you can be the second opinion.

• Discuss the purpose of a hospital. As you ask women why they prefer hospitals for birth, you can present the idea that hospitals are for illness and problems. Our first goal should be to birth at home, unassisted. The second option should be a midwife-assisted birth, provided there are competent midwives available. The next option should be a doctor-assisted hospital birth. The last resort for birth should be a high technology, doctor-directed event.

• Avoid drugs during labor and delivery because: (1) they are unsafe; (2) they interfere with the brain-body chemistry before, during and after birth; (3) they affect immediate breastfeeding success; (4) they decrease the likelihood of a pleasurable birth release; (5) they affect the alertness and energy level of the mother and baby; (6) they affect postpartum attachment and bonding.

• Discuss the five standards of safe childbearing and the importance of having standards. The five standards as presented by David Stewart are: nutrition, natural birth, homebirth, breastfeeding and skillful midwifery. Those who birth in the absence of trained medical providers act as their own midwives or attendants. Dialogue about safety would be especially helpful with skeptical friends and relatives. The greatest impact you make might be with your most passionate, but open-minded opponent.

• Teach your daughter (and son) about fertility and birth control. Your knowledge of fertility will improve as you teach someone else. Mastery and comfort with our childbearing power enables us to make intelligent decisions. Gratitude and awe towards pregnancy, childbearing and childrearing are more likely when pregnancy is surrounded by natural methods.

Mastery in a subject area enables better decision-making and smart decisions are part of responsible, mature adulthood. Your children can share this information with their partners. We are inundated with information about artificial contraception, but not with natural methods. Even if you are not interested in natural methods, your children will be in a better position to make decisions about their reproductive health if they were presented with all of the options. Parents who present an honest, positive attitude about sex, life and birth will have a better chance raising children who respect sex, birth and family life.

• Sponsor an "alternative" bridal or baby shower. Encourage people to give gifts of service rather than material presents. Coordinate a program or facilitate a discussion at the shower. Depending on the needs of those present, some topics could include: risks and reliability of birth control, breast self-exams, menopause, marriage, pregnancy, birth and breastfeeding, infections and disease, eating and exercise, hysterectomies, community resources of supportive people.

• Create an alternative birth handbook. List local OB/Gyns, pediatricians, chiropractors, other doctors, midwives, childbirth educators, lactation consultants and any individual or group that supports unassisted homebirth, natural childbirth, breastfeeding and attachment parenting. Include magazines and resources, as well as brief information on homeschooling, home-based businesses, natural health or large family living. Identify problem people in your community. For example, if you are opposed to abortion, C-sections, circumcisions or immunizations, create a list of those who aggressively support these options, and update it annually and make the list easily accessible to women in your community.

• Determine needs in your area so that you can help improve, expose or commend some practices. Encourage a local crisis pregnancy center to conduct periodic surveys asking doctors and hospitals such things as C-section and abortion rates. Gather information from the state birth and death certificate records department. On the bottom of many birth certificate forms is an area where doctors complete information about prenatal care, including how many ultrasounds the mother had and how many weeks her pregnancy lasted.

• Be a change agent for hospital births. Perhaps you can help women who choose traditional methods to have a better birth: suggest women to give birth while standing or squatting; advise women to touch and breastfeed the baby immediately after birth; encourage women to watch the pediatrician perform newborn exams.

• Form an unassisted homebirth support group. List your phone number at the library, with childbirth educators or La Leche League. You may never have a meeting or serve any purpose except for others to contact you. In our area, DIY families get together a few times a year for an informal, potluck cookout. DIYers are included in a Homebirth Education Network facilitated by a midwife.

• Volunteer and get involved in childbirth education, and be a constant example to others. Because of you, someone might refuse another scheduled C-section or epidural and opt for a certified nurse-midwife attendant at a birthing center. As long as women take more responsibility and feel a greater sense of autonomy, they will have greater satisfaction about their births and being new mothers. Women on Level Four of *The Birth Pyramid* especially need help.

• Donate books or magazine subscriptions to your local library. Some libraries may allow you to insert a sticker on the back jacket which identifies the donor. What a perfect opportunity to list that group you started!

• Write letters to the editor when an opportunity presents itself and be sure to write television producers commending good births or criticizing stereotypical births.

• Refuse health coverage that does not support your philosophies. Choose or persuade insurance companies to reimburse midwife-assisted homebirths and alternative care. Some insurance plans offer home visits for newborn care. Consumer spending habits need to change so that the providers will make changes.

Those who wish to be publicly outspoken about homebirth may want to go beyond the role of educating, mentoring, and advocating unassisted homebirth. It may be important to exert some effort to ensure that unassisted homebirth remains legal. Do not underestimate the power of networking. Encourage one of your birth advocate friends to keep abreast of the legal issues surrounding unassisted homebirth or homebirth in general because there may be a time when DIY birthers might want to join forces. Many people want to outlaw and regulate midwife-assisted homebirths. It is unfortunate that a segment of the population is intolerant of a couple's choice to have a baby according to their desires, especially since midwifery has had successful results.

Rather than fight proponents of unassisted homebirth and midwife-assisted homebirth, we should seek cooperation by encouraging partnerships between doctors and couples and between lay midwives and hospitals.

Thriving, not just surviving, is our birthright as women. Do not cringe and make yourself small if you are called the black sheep, the maverick, the lone wolf. Those with slow seeing say a nonconformist is a blight on society. But it has been proven over the centuries, that being different means standing at the edge, means one is practically guaranteed to make an original contribution, a useful and stunning contribution to her culture. —Clarissa Pinkola Estes

PART VI

Birth Stories: Putting it all Together

The stories in this book are from births which occurred in the 1990's. The path each couple takes on their birth journey is very different. The following stories show us the many ways of birthing. Each story is different, yet couples end up in the same place: a place of personal discovery and a greater love within their families.

19

Unplanned Unassisted Birth

Matthew and Wendy Bunkelman
Monroe, MI
Not a Moment to Spare

After 1-1/2 hours of labor, Abigail Li was born on October 24, 1995. The midwives did not make it on time for the birth and Matt returned home just minutes before the baby was born.

Our birth story begins in March of 1995 when my husband Matthew and I discovered that I was pregnant again. Carly, our eldest daughter, was born just nine months prior and was completely breastfed. We were surprised, yet joyous upon learning the good news. The next nine months were spent looking forward to our homebirth with a midwife.

Even though Carly's birth was an unintervened, unmedicated birth, I knew that the hospital was not where I was meant to give birth; it just didn't feel right. Matt and I started our quest for a midwife. Our prayers were answered and we were wonderfully surprised to find some loving, Christian women, who believed and trusted in the miracle of birth, and who agreed to help us achieve our birth at home.

As the months progressed, I felt so wonderful, so full of life. I took pride in my pregnancy and my growing belly and I felt so beautiful. I absorbed myself into books on homebirth and midwifery. I sensed that this birth was going to be different from my last. Carly was born after a precipitous labor, so I prayed diligently that this birth would be longer. I hoped for an easier transition for my baby to life outside of my womb and I had to trust that this would be a less intense experience for me also. Little did I know that this was not God's plan for our homebirth.

Three weeks before my due date, I started experiencing some contractions. They were coming pretty regularly, but were not too uncomfortable. After a glass of wine and a hot bath, they dissipated. We resolved that it was "false labor" and persevered on for another week.

On October 24, after what seemed to be a long and very restless evening of sleep, my daughter and I awoke to the most beautiful autumn morning ever. The sun filled the bedroom, and as we laid together in bed, Carly at my breast, I felt a very fierce sensation in my belly and knew instinctively that today was to be our birth day. I was feeling confident and ready for the day we had so eagerly anticipated. After I lost my mucous plug, I gave Matt a "buzz" at work.

By 9:00 A.M. my contractions were 20-30 seconds long, coming about every three minutes. I sensed that I should call Barbara, our midwife, as I was feeling a little confused and overwhelmed by the power of these contractions. She said she was on her way. Shortly after that phone call, I found myself having to concentrate more on each contraction. I was unable to care for Carly, and after dropping several eggs on the floor trying to make breakfast, I decided to call my mother-in-law, who was planning to watch Carly during the birth. Mary Ann arrived ten minutes later and I retreated to my bedroom to labor alone.

My contractions had become quite powerful. I leaned against my bed, and sitting on my knees, I withdrew deep into my being where my breath became my focus and my body opened. Moments (but what seemed like centuries) later I realized that my times of quiet between contractions had become shorter. In fact, the contractions were one on top of the other.

"Where is Matt," I thought, "Oh, God. Am I going to have this baby by myself?" It was at this time that I decided to take a hot bath, anything to slow this labor down. I just kept thinking that I had to wait for Matt. I could not have this baby without Matt. *You can do it!*

It was in the bathtub that I had my first strong urge to push, and so just as I jumped onto the toilet, Matt walked into the front door. "Short breaths," Matt kept saying to me. "Just keep breathing." He was sure that this birth would wait for the midwives. But soon, my whole body took over and pushing my baby out was all I could do. "Matt. It's coming! The baby is coming." I felt her move down through the birth canal and I intuitively jumped off of the toilet to hang onto the side of the tub and moaned. I think that Matt was experiencing a brief moment of denial before he realized that the baby was coming and the midwives were not.

hat a great birth ut - her

Then, as though he had done it 100 times before, he calmly helped me to birth our baby. As her head crowned, my water broke, and with two more pushes Abigail's body slid out of mine and into her father's loving arms. Nothing could have been more miraculous than that moment in time.

Unexpectedly, Abbey let out a beautiful cry and Carly exclaimed from the living room, "A baby!" Matt passed Abigail through my legs and as I held her little body close to mine we walked together to the bedroom. We wrapped her in blankets and while we laid together in bed nursing, Abbey's curious sister and proud grandmother came in to welcome her into our tender world.

Abigail Li's birth was not my "ideal birth." The entire birth was 1-1/2 hours long. It was violent, exasperating really. But I was so astonished and I still am today of the love that I felt: love for myself, love for my husband, and love for the baby that slept contentedly in my adoring arms.

so sweet!

Frank and Kim Pratt
Pasadena, MD
Where on Earth is our Midwife?

Kim's labor progressed so quickly that her midwife was not able to make it for the birth. Alana was born into her father's hands on June 5, 1996.

On June 5th, I was a little past my due date. I was very huge and uncomfortable and decided to take some castor oil. It was 9:00 A.M., my husband Frank was at work and I was feeling a little nervous because I didn't know what to expect. About an hour later, I called Frank and asked him to come home. I wasn't feeling anything, but I wanted him with me anyway.

Frank came home and played with our son Gannon while I washed about five loads of laundry and hung them on the clothesline. We went to the park and I walked a good bit. I kept getting these bands of pain around my back and lower abdomen, but ignored them because I thought they were from the castor oil. I told Frank I wanted to be at home, so we left. We stopped at a produce stand on the way home and bought some sunflowers to plant.

I took a four hour nap when we got home and continued to ignore the bands of pain. I woke up to find that my water broke. Frank was outside playing with our two year old son, Gannon, and I called him in. I told him to call our midwife and let her know that my water broke. I went into the bathroom to wash the sticky, amniotic fluid off my legs.

Frank was talking to our midwife and I got on to tell her what happened. She didn't seem to think that the baby would be born that fast and said she would wait fifteen minutes before getting on the road. She lived 45 minutes away. Frank asked me what he could do and I told him to clean the bathroom while I made the bed.

While making the bed, I had a killer contraction. I went over to the toilet and was feeling restless. I asked Frank to call our friend and while he was on the phone, I had a massive contraction and thought to myself, "I can't take another one of these." Frank got off the phone and continued cleaning the bathroom. As I went to sit on the toilet, I told him I had to push. He said, "No, don't push," and I said, "I have to." *your body knows what to do*

I got on the bed and was trying to hold back my urge to push. Realizing that he would probably be delivering our baby, Frank came in and said, "I can do this. I've washed my hands." He gave me a pep talk about how we can do this and to just trust him. I remember thinking, "I know we can do this."

Pushing this baby was a lot harder than the first. Finally, her head came out. Frank told me, "Okay, push! We have to get her body out." I said, "No." I just didn't feel like pushing anymore. When I did finally push the baby out, Frank laid the baby on my belly and covered her. My friend showed up and let the dog and poor little Gannon in, who was pounding on the back door yelling, "Momma, are you okay?" We originally planned on him witnessing the birth, but it didn't work out that way.

A short while later the midwife showed up. Frank finally got to cut the cord. The midwife weighed Alana who was a whopping 9 lbs.! The midwife and her apprentice cleaned up as I showered. I was very touched when my friend stayed with me in the bathroom to make sure that I didn't fall down or anything.

When I came out, the bed was made which was so nice. Alana was good at nursing from the start. I couldn't believe how calm and quiet she was. After our midwife, apprentice and friend left, we marveled at our new, sweet, little girl.

When everyone found out that we had an unassisted homebirth, they hailed Frank as some sort of hero. It really made me angry, as if I wasn't even there. I was proud of Frank, but also proud of myself. My body made a perfect person and birthed a perfect person. Birth is a big mystery, but it is also the most natural thing a woman can do. Women have done it for thousands of years. No one thinks of the woman's body as being the miracle it is. Whoever the person was who

WTF! people!

you're the one that birthed your baby. not Frank!

ugh!

simply caught the baby is the one who is respected. It doesn't make sense to me. *me either!*

As of this writing, Alana is eight months old. She is still a gentle and sweet little thing, although not so quiet anymore. She has to yell over her big brother who has finally adjusted to the trauma of having a new person to share his mommy and daddy with. I'd like to have another baby, definitely at home!

20

Young Lovers

Keith and Cindy Earley-Steinke
Lynchburg, VA
A Family Birth

Even though Cindy's knowledge and experience of childbirth surpasses others, she encountered hostility and arrogance from the medical community for her birth decision. Ultimately none of that matters. The unassisted homebirth produced a new dimension in their marriage and a lovely daughter, Corrine, who was born on October 24, 1996.

Our first daughter was born in a hospital with a certified nurse-midwife in attendance. It was a great birth experience, but we were not happy with the hospital stay. Before we were pregnant the second time we had decided on a homebirth, and on the heels of that, an unattended one. Our former midwife wasn't allowed to attend homebirths and we weren't happy with the local choices, as limited as they were. We originally planned on having other people at the birth, but eventually decided against that as well. I felt that because of my position as a childbirth educator, I would be expected to live up to some ideal of behavior during labor. I didn't want to feel as though I was "performing" for anyone. I didn't want the stress of worrying about "doing things right." I wanted to be free to cry, moan, or "give up" and know that my husband would understand everything. I knew from the first birth that <u>when I would say</u> "I can't do this anymore," he would say, "I know you can," and there wouldn't be any panic.

I don't agree with the belief that some midwife is better than no midwife. If you have significantly different philosophies or ideas about how things should go, then the possible tension that could arise during the birth far outweighs the possible benefit, especially when the mother in question is <u>healthy, well prepared, and well informed.</u> Everything was going great during the pregnancy, but we had decided to have an attendant if it turned out there were twins or the baby was breech. We eventually ruled out both scenarios even though I still had this nagging feeling there might be two in there.

It was a Wednesday night and I had just finished teaching one of my classes. My students were leaving and wished me luck on going into labor soon. I was 41 weeks along. I said, "Maybe tonight," but I had no feeling one way or the other. I nursed our daughter (30 months old) to sleep in our bed around 11:30 P.M. and my husband fell asleep shortly thereafter. I was reading and relaxing when suddenly I felt and heard a pop and a snap near my pubic bone. The clock said 12:30 A.M. and I decided to see what would happen next. Suddenly, I coughed and my pants were wet.

I woke my husband and told him to wash out the crock pot (for hot compresses) and then told him he could go back to sleep. Contractions started in five minutes and continued to be five minutes apart. <u>Relaxing through them was so much easier this time</u>. Around 1:00 A.M. I got up to get in the tub and my husband started gathering the supplies in the living room. I helped Keith for a while and then started soaking.

Around 2:00 A.M. we debated about waking up a neighbor to come over and take videos. We wanted to have a permanent, tangible record of the birth, but we also wanted to be alone. Being alone won out! Keith asked if I was going to get out of the tub, but I knew if I did that I'd start walking and things would really start picking up. Boy did they! Immediately contractions were one minute apart and I was in transition. One minute I was freezing, the next minute hot, and always very thirsty! I'm not one who likes to be touched much in labor, but just Keith's <u>presence and voice</u> comforted me.

At this point, we lost a little confidence. It was about 3:30 A.M. and I had been through transition. I felt I should be ready to push, but I didn't have an overwhelming urge to do so. We both tried checking dilation, unsuccessfully! However, the peaks of contractions were painful and I could no longer relax or stay put during them. This should have been a big clue, but I think I was in denial. Even though our first baby was a four hour labor, I still didn't believe it could be happening this fast. That is when I first started saying, "I can't do this anymore."

Around 5:00 A.M. I decided to push anyway. Keith said he could see the head descending, so I told him to go ahead and wake up Celeste. Then it seemed as if no progress was being made, and I soon regretted having Celeste awake so soon. She was sitting across from me and kept asking, "What are you doing Mommy?" "I'm having a baby Punkin'," I'd reply. Then she noticed a moth flying around one of the lamps. "A bug Daddy! A bug! A bug! A bug!" she was screaming. Keith looked at me helpless. Should he attend to me or her? "Get the damn bug," I whispered. *haha!*

I decided to get into the tub once again. It had helped in Celeste's birth, but then I only pushed for eight minutes with her. As soon as I was submerged, Corinne's head did a rapid descent. I couldn't move my legs far enough apart in our little tub, but I told Keith, "It's coming now!" "Are we having a waterbirth?" he asked. "Not by choice," I replied. The descent stopped long enough for me to get out and move to my nest in the living room. As soon as I squatted, she started crowning.

Keith applied <u>hot compresses and pressure</u> to my perineum. Once her head emerged, he felt for the cord and informed me it was there. I asked him if he could get it (we had clamps just in case) and he said to hold off a little. "I can't!" I breathed, but I must have because he had time to unwind it twice. It's funny because we had practiced this very same scenario with a baby doll and shoestring! When her body emerged, we lifted her up together. Out of the corner of my eye, I noticed Celeste watching in astonishment. As much preparation as she had had, I don't think she believed a baby was ever going to come. Keith and I were half crying, half laughing with joy. Celeste came over and touched the new baby. It was several minutes before we even cared to check the sex.

Corinne started nursing in five minutes and the placenta came out in 10-15 minutes. I was on the phone with my mom when a contraction came on and I felt my abdomen. It was so hard that I was sure I was feeling another backbone! I told my mom, "I gotta go. I'm either pushing out another baby or the placenta!" We waited almost thirty minutes to cut the cord, and even then we saw no need to clamp it. We used an herbal dust for the stump and it healed and fell off in four days. She weighed 8 lbs. 4 oz. (1 oz. less than her sister) and was 21 inches long. There were no perineal tears, just as before.

Having her at home, and unattended, gave me such a feeling of pride and accomplishment; yet at the same time I knew we hadn't done anything that the majority of healthy, informed couples couldn't do. There was such a feeling of continuity and wholeness—no disruption or break in our lives. I strongly feel that this accounts for Celeste's acceptance of Corinne (that and tandem nursing!). I definitely feel closer to and more in love with my husband. We had had some trust issues in the past and this birth definitely healed some old hurts. He is my lover, my partner, my rock.

Would we do it this way again? Only with a few small changes. First, I'd like to have a better back-up plan in case of a complication, namely a midwife on call. We were depending on an ambulance and complete unannounced transference this time. Second, my husband owns his own business and he was right in the middle of a job. We agreed that he should go on in and we had his mother come over to help clean up and do things for me. I deeply regret this now. We both feel he should have stayed home that day so we could all just lay around and bond. It was a very dumb decision in hindsight.

Third, I took Shepherd's Purse in case I was hemorrhaging (I bleed a lot anyway, so it's hard to tell). Later I developed an infection due to a retained piece of amniotic sac, and I wonder if that was the cause. My reasoning is that the midwife who treated me told me that the doctor she's in practice with had a patient with the same problem. I think he regularly administers Pitocin for the expulsion of the placenta. I didn't take the remedy until after the placenta was out, but I wonder if, as a vasoconstrictor, it caused a clamping down that didn't allow the piece to pass.

I was thrilled with the birth and thrilled with not having outsiders there. Being alone for the birth seemed to create a magical aura around the house. Someone else, anyone else, would have broken that spell. There was a special excitement that only we were sharing. It was like waking up in the middle of the night and sneaking off with your spouse to make love by the fireplace. You wouldn't call anyone over for that, would you? Having done this makes us realize that we can do anything we set our minds to.

My husband and I communicate better and are closer. I also felt like resuming sex sooner this time even though the first birth was completely natural and there were no tears or anything. The only difference between the births was location and attendant. Nothing bonds a couple like sharing the intimate moment of birth. I'm sure the experience also explains the closeness between Celeste and her new baby sister. At 5:40 A.M. on October 24th, 1996, Corinne Marianna made this world a little bit better place to be.

Michael and Allison Scimeca
Atlanta, Georgia
Unconditional Faith

Allison and Michael are proof that birth is not only a beautiful love encounter, but that it can be pleasurable. After spending 30 hours in labor, a 100 lb. woman gives birth to her first baby, 8-1/5 lb. Anthony on August 14, 1993. Then on February 1, 1996, their second DIY brought forth Angela.

"Unconditional faith" was the theme of my whole pregnancy and labor. This was my first child and I did not know what to expect. I just followed my intuition and knew I was protected by God. I read *Birth and the Dialogue of Love* many times and it was that book that I used for guidance in preparing for a homebirth. The love and support my husband Michael gave me throughout my labor was incredible. I would have never had the same care with anyone else because no one can care for me the way my husband can. I was relaxed and comfortable and the mood was perfect.

After labor began, Michael and I took a shower together. From then on we stayed naked. He began massaging my perineum with such care and intent that I knew I was in competent hands. We sang together, stared in each others eyes, talked, ate, and slept for two hours. Before I knew it, thirty hours had elapsed and our son was born. It was the ultimate climax. I felt open, loose and free.

Words cannot explain the feeling as my baby's body slithered out. To this day, I can still sense that wonderful feeling inside. It makes me tingle. I weigh only 100 pounds and our baby was 8-1/5 pounds, according to the bathroom scale. I did not rip at all.

Many people commented on how alert, perceptive and aware Anthony John was as an infant and it was very obvious to me that this was indeed true. I believe the way we welcomed him into the world was solely responsible for this. From conception to birth, I was surrounded with love and faith that childbirth is a most beautiful and natural process and now I know from experience that this is definitely true.

Having contractions five minutes apart for most of the thirty hours of labor, I can only imagine what they would have done to me if I were in the hospital. I believe God always knows what is best and therefore choose to never interfere with His intelligence.

My husband and I decided to have another unassisted homebirth with the arrival of Angela Jule. This time we were hoping to have Anthony with us, who was 2-1/2. We prepared him well for the event. We had undress rehearsals and continually educated him on what to expect.

This pregnancy was different from my first. My husband and I were more intimately connected with each other. With Anthony's birth, we learned to trust nature as we surrendered to what was a thirty hour labor. This time we were more physically active and did less observing and more participating. I was a lot more educated with Angela's birth. For instance, I studied the three stages of labor in depth. With Anthony, I had little knowledge of the stages. I also explored myself and was more in tune with my physical and emotional feelings. The connection to my husband was obvious as I was able to openly express exactly what I was feeling. I visualized the way the baby was lying inside me and felt deeply connected with her, realizing we were two different humans although bonded together in a relationship that will never end.

Two weeks before I went into labor, I was in the bathtub and could feel her head internally. It was an amazing feeling knowing that I had a fully developed person inside me and that we were only separated by tissue.

We were all just waiting. On January 31st, I woke up with a burst of energy. That evening I put Anthony to bed at 9:30 P.M. after reading a story to him. I got up ten minutes later and instantly felt a warm sensation in my lower back. It felt like a big hand was holding onto my tailbone, a familiar feeling I had during my first labor. "This could be the night," I said to Michael when I called him at work. I tried to lay down to get some rest but was too excited. It was now 10:00 P.M. and the sensations were getting stronger. At 10:30, the sensations inspired me to squat up against the couch. I experienced an energy that was not a contraction, but very pleasurable. At the same time my husband came home and saw that I was totally tuned in with myself. We hung around downstairs for about an hour and a half packing our picnic and gathering anything else we might need. We knew that once we went upstairs to our bedroom we were not going to come back down.

Since our first labor took thirty hours, we took our time getting ready. I came out of the bathroom feeling things were moving along real fast and had yet to prepare our bed with plastic sheets or cover the pillows. The sensations were more stronger and frequent. When the sensations came, I felt my actions were well orchestrated. At times I sat up, rocked back and forth, hummed, concentrated on connecting to my breath, and relaxed.

When my husband joined me in an aroma oil bath, the love between us became apparent. When we got out of the tub we went straight to the bed. I went and stayed on all fours. Michael got underneath me and we kissed and caressed each other. At times he would rub my back. We even had intercourse and we both were reaching climax when I felt the baby right there.

I had an urge to go to the bathroom. As I sat on the toilet, I had my first real contraction. It was big, strong, intense and pleasurable. As I hung onto Michael's shoulders, I had another one. It felt so great to just hang there and have gravity weigh me down. I had another contraction and this time actually felt the baby rapidly drop down into the birth canal. I reached down and to my surprise felt the head.

We walked over to the bed where I had Michael perform perineal massage. I held back the baby's head. I did not want to rip. "Lubricate me. This baby is going to fly out." On the fourth contraction the head came out. I felt this enormous build up of pressure inside. It was the water that never broke. When her head was out I could feel her kicking inside of me. I knew that I was building up to an ultimate climax and was anxious for the release. Another contraction came but only her arm popped out. My husband felt her neck to make sure the cord wasn't wrapped around it. As he did that, I had another contraction. Wow!

Out she came along with the amniotic fluid. My husband was caught up in the emotional beauty of the whole event as I had the biggest, sexiest orgasmic release of my life. He was crying and I was panting. We looked at the clock and could not believe it was only 2:10 A.M. I sat up on the bed. My placenta came out right away. Our baby immediately nursed for twenty minutes on each breast. At 4:00 A.M. we cut the cord and by 4:30 A.M. we were snuggled up in bed with our precious Angela Jule beside us.

"Boy, does our son have a surprise to wake up to in the morning," I thought. We closed our eyes and fell asleep thinking of the miracle that we had created through an act of love that was now complete.

Expression and communication in the peak-experiences tend often to become poetic, mythical and rhapsodic, as if this were the natural kind of language to express such states of being. —Abraham Maslow

There is only one way to keep the relationship "vital and growing"—intimate, husband/wife homebirthing.
—Marilyn Moran

21

Spirit-Led Birth

Troy and Shannon McNear
Goose Creek, SC
Faith and Trust

After three hospital births, Shannon was looking forward to a DIY birth. Born in Zion and All the Way Home had a profound impact upon her. Her commitment to homebirth intensified. Unwilling to bend to "the rules" (most of them arbitrary) of the system and a desire for a deeper spiritual and emotional experience became a reality with the birth of Ross on December 16, 1995.

Ross was born into his daddy's waiting hands, while I knelt next to our bed, with a close friend assisting. The very fact that he was my largest baby (10 lbs. 3 oz.), was to me a witness that it was God's power at work. I had a tiny tear because the delivery was so quick. Some things were unexpected: I thought that sitting in the tub to ease the pain would help but it didn't.

I was fighting a battle with fear—fear of pain, not that anything would go wrong. When I got to the point where I started saying, "I can't," then I felt the Lord gently urging me to call on His name during the contractions. So began this litany of praise which incredibly carried me through the contractions when nothing else seemed to be working. I would not have felt comfortable doing that in a hospital with a doctor and strange nurses present! There was something unique about praising God in spite of the pain.

One highlight during labor was a moment which gave me a burst of excitement. Troy was unpacking the birth supplies, snapped up the receiving blanket, and shouted, "Baby!" That to me embodied his enthusiasm for the birth and I'll never forget it! Once we made the decision, he embraced it with determination and joy.

It was beautiful to see my husband accepting and shouldering the *spiritual* responsibility, both of us as one and trusting God to give me a safe delivery. There has been a new tenderness between us since Ross' birth. I feel that God has worked a healing of sorts in our relationship. I realized during my pregnancy that I had never really trusted Troy as the head of our household. Even when I thought I was being submissive, I had still resented him for past hurts and failures.

For me, the birth was trusting that God could and would work through Troy as my most immediate authority, and guide the birth by his hands. The joy and gratitude that most women exude after birth belongs to their husbands and to God, not to some doctor. I learned that even though I may not see Troy growing as quickly as I would like, I also have a lot of learning to do.

In all, I was just awestruck over the whole thing, as I know most homebirth parents must be. And the awe lingers, not just over the birth itself, but how we came to our present, somewhat extreme position, from three hospital births, two of which were inductions, to a "medically unattended" homebirth. Since reading *The Way Home* after my first baby, I've longed for a homebirth, but finally learned that it probably wasn't going to happen for us unless we just committed to it and exercised some real faith.

We tried with our second baby, but wound up going with a doctor in the last month. With our third child, we didn't want to pay a midwife only to end up in a hospital. I think homebirth is like breastfeeding—you can't just try it, you have to just do it. Between seeing the way a couple of my friends were treated when they had their babies—things which we felt in our hearts were wrong, but we could not prove—and a book or two which the Lord sent our way, by the time we conceived this baby, the Lord had prepared us for a homebirth, even if we had to do it ourselves. They call it "do-it-yourself" homebirth. Who's really doing it anyway? Does a doctor bring this baby out, or the Lord? It just seems like a revelation when you discover it for yourself.

Bill and Jeanie Haas
Bear Creek, PA
New Beginnings

The Haas' have the courage to face that which is within themselves: their fears, their sufferings, their weaknesses. Their four DIYs began with the birth of Emily on December 8, 1988. Anna was born on November 8, 1991 and then came Matthew on November 11, 1994. Abigail, the youngest Haas, was born on April 1, 1996.

Our decision to homebirth was not a sudden one. We had a daughter born by C-section in November, 1981. Although we were thrilled to have a healthy baby, we were very disappointed with the birth experience. Not only was the section unnecessary, I was anesthetized and my husband was not allowed to be there. Many things were not as we had been told they would be.

For our second child, we found a doctor willing to allow me a VBAC. The year was 1984 and VBACs had not been as common as they are today. I was so thrilled I would deliver naturally that I didn't mind being in the hospital. I strongly disliked the machines and internal exams, but was willing to succumb to it as long as I didn't have to have another C-section.

By the time our third child was due, I dreaded the thought of going to a hospital. Still, we were not ready to deliver at home. I was in active labor upon arrival to the hospital, but was so uncomfortable that my labor slowed way down. I finally delivered and insisted on going home that day. I could hardly wait to get home!

During my fourth pregnancy, we decided that we really wanted a homebirth. We wrote down every Bible verse that we could find that pertained to childbirth. We saturated our hearts and minds with God's word until we had a deep peace that things would be fine. I don't think we would have had a baby at home if there were any doubts about safety. We truly believe that home is safer, especially for the one who is trusting God.

We ordered birth supplies through *Spirit-Led Childbirth* catalog and awaited the big day. Looking back, I see that we acted in simple faith and it was a wonderful experience. The nicest thing was being able to labor naturally and listen to my body.

I'll never forget when my water broke. I looked at my friend and said, "Something just happened. I think my water broke." This was my fourth delivery, yet I never experienced my water breaking because it had always been broken for me! My labor and delivery were uneventful, but so joyful. It felt so right being at home. We are convinced that God intended babies to be born into the arms of their loving "daddy-midwives."

Since Emily's homebirth was such a wonderful, peaceful, faith-building experience, we eagerly awaited our second homebirth almost three years later. On the morning of November 8, 1991, my labor began with what is commonly called "bloody show," or losing one's mucous plug. Throughout the day, I had mild contractions. By eight o'clock that evening, I called our pastor's wife, Margie, who would be helping with the birth, and asked her to come. Bill put our other four children to bed and it was peaceful and quiet.

By ten o'clock, contractions were strong and I experienced occasional nausea. Since nausea was a part of my previous labors during transition, I had a bowl nearby. I remember that moist, very warm cloths (we used cotton diapers) felt *wonderful* draped across my belly. Labor progressed quickly, and by 10:30 I thought I had to have a bowel movement. The "bowel movement" turned out to be a baby. My water broke as she came down the birth canal. It all happened so quickly. I remember asking, "What in the world kind of labor was that?"

Margie and Bill cleaned up and awaited my placenta. After Emily's birth in 1988, the placenta did not expel for twelve hours and we were hopeful that it would not take as long this time. I was settled in nursing and we decided that Margie could return to her family. Bill left to tend to a child or get some rest and a few minutes later, my body began a "second labor." For the next two or three hours, I had incredibly hard contractions which seemed more difficult because I was alone and out of earshot of my husband. These contractions were totally unexpected. Finally, sometime early in the morning, my placenta delivered and the contractions stopped. I was finally able to settle down with our new little blessing and sleep.

Later, Bill and Margie felt awful when they heard what I had been through, but we considered it a learning experience. When attending a birth or giving birth, I make sure someone is with the birth mom until the placenta has delivered.

On November 11, 1994, I had a DIY with the same helpers. It was uneventful, but longer than expected. Our little boy was born in the water bag, which is easily pulled away. Bill said that it disintegrates. Sadly, our son was born with a congenital heart malformation and lived for only one month. When I conceived again within six months, I experienced bittersweet emotions. I was thrilled to be pregnant, but had a lot of fear to deal with.

I wrestled with God for several months, thinking, "Anything for you, God, but just don't let another baby die!" Two experiences brought me peace. Once, while weeping during a worship service, I felt God telling me he was going to bless me. Shortly after that, I was reading my Bible when a verse was "highlighted" for me; "I will perfect that which concerns you." This was during my fifth month and those words settled into my heart. I knew that whatever I faced, God would be there to help. I was at peace and felt that all would be fine.

The pregnancy proceeded well. However, during the last six weeks, I felt a tingly feeling in my hands. I think this was partly pressure from the baby as well as retained, excess fluid. I was not as careful as I should have been about my diet, particularly my sugar intake. Margie was not able to help at this birth and we knew a midwife who agreed to come. She lived 1-1/2 hours away. On March 31st, my husband's birthday, labor began with mild contractions. By evening, the contractions were stronger, so we called the midwife. We were informed that our midwife was out of town and that her daughter/assistant was available to attend our birth. We hung up, thought about it, and when we called back, she told us she had another woman in labor and couldn't leave. She suggested coming to her home, but we didn't want to do that.

My husband said that he would be the "midwife" and we settled in for what turned out to be a long haul! I continued having irregular, weak contractions throughout the night and next day. By the next evening, I was feeling the urge to push, but the baby was high. I could feel kicking high in my chest. Because I have never had to push for a long time, I began to feel a little nervous and anxious, wondering why nothing seemed to be happening. I was restless; I sat on the birthing stool, climbed back in bed and sat on the rocking chair.

My husband knew I was battling anxiety and told our daughter to get his Scripture cards. As he began to read the Bible verses to me, I felt hope and encouragement. Our little girl was born within minutes! One funny note: When my husband saw her head, he said, "Push. Keep pushing," and the baby just flew out. She was born in the water bag, which Bill peeled away. I kept waiting for my water to break, which probably added to my concern. My placenta delivered normally, for which I was very thankful. Abigail was 9 lbs. 8 oz., strong and healthy. Our oldest daughter, 14 year-old Sarah, served as my husband's apprentice.

22

Large Happy Families

Bert and Sheila Stubbs
Strathroy, Ontario, Canada
Flesh of my Flesh

The Stubbs have six children. Their first hospital birth was a C-section, followed by a vaginal delivery. The next two children were delivered at home by a General Practitioner. The last two were born into their father's hands at home, with the General Practitioner observing the birth of the sixth child.

The birth of our fifth child was an unplanned DIY, sort of. I had mentioned to Bert several times that it would be nice giving birth to him, not some doctor. "Wouldn't it be nice if the doctor wasn't here at all?" "Don't even think of it!" was Bert's response. Much to my surprise, I was in labor in less than 24 hours. I was a month early!

I woke up at 2:00 A.M. with contractions and didn't bother to call the doctor. I didn't wake Bert up until I was getting very uncomfortable. We got a few supplies ready, very few. We got the towels out, covered the floor with plastic, then called the doctor. I said there was no hurry. Then, knowing I was ready and the doctor would be coming soon, I suddenly found myself pushing. I was calm, quiet, relaxed and thrilled that my baby was coming on its own time.

I had never had an urge to push before, but was always told when to, even when I didn't want to. The baby slipped out so quickly. Bert was scared and begged me not to push. "Will you just shut up!" I said. He was holding me and I didn't realize that I was pushing. I sat on the floor and he saw the baby's head. I laugh when I think of how he kept saying, "What do I do? What do I do?" And he was doing it!

In spite of this lovely birth, when we were pregnant with our sixth child, Bert did not want to do it alone again. He was too nervous being solely responsible. A friend came over to help out, but knowing how I felt, stayed out while the baby was being born. If only I could get the doctor to do the same. His presence irritated me even though he stayed by the door. He wanted to check me and I wouldn't let him. He wanted me in a different position and I refused. I didn't like him watching me any more than I'd want him watching me have sex, use the toilet, or take a bath. Having had a DIY, I had something to compare a private birth with a doctor-attended birth.

When the baby was finally born after much pushing, the doctor got immediately busy tying and cutting the cord. That's when I really noticed the intrusion. The first moments after the DIY of our fifth child were so romantic, but this time, procedure got in the way. I even think my pushing stage would have been easier without him watching.

I might consider a hospital birth again, if they'd leave you alone. It would never happen; they like to use their techno-toys.

Patricia and Rick Kohl
Hopkinton, NY
Our Autumn Blessing

The Kohl's have seven children, two of which were DIY births. Timothy was born on July 22, 1992 and Pauline was welcomed into the family on September 18, 1996.

Our sixth baby, Timothy Peter, was born into his daddy's hands on July 22, 1992 after a seven-hour labor. This was our first do it yourself birth. Our first, Regina, was born in a hospital in Hawaii, after which I said "Never again in a hospital," and I was a registered nurse. The next four children, Gretchen, Valerie, Conrad and Genevieve were all born at home with midwives. All the homebirths were good births without any medical interventions and all the midwives were very lovely, caring ladies.

When I read the information that Marilyn Moran had sent me after seeing her ad in a childbirth book, it made me realize that we could have a still much better birth with the intimacy of just husband and wife present. But Rick and I were still unsure if we had the courage to give birth unassisted.

We contacted one of the two midwives in our area and went to see her. She discussed with me mostly things I already knew and her fee for attending the birth was more than we could afford. I am Rh negative and she would do no blood work. Rick and I discussed the matter almost daily and prayed to do the right thing. Deep down I knew that I wanted to be alone with my husband to give birth. During this time, Marilyn Moran sent us the book, *Happy Birth Days*. This cemented my desire and courage for this type of birth. After Rick read it, he had no more qualms about delivering his own child. We had made our decision and were now at peace. I called and canceled the midwife.

As for prenatal care, I did it all myself (good diet, rest, good vitamins, herbal tinctures and teas specific for pregnancy, blood pressure and urine checks). I did visit a doctor once, about a month before I was due so that he could check the position of the baby and do an antibody blood test. He agreed to back us up should the need for medical assistance arise, and for that I am most grateful. We did not tell him that we were doing unassisted, and he didn't ask.

I went into labor at 6:30 A.M., three days past my due date. I awoke in the morning with a slight bloody show and very mild contractions. We called our good friends who came and got our four youngest children. Regina, our 17 year-old, stayed to help with various tasks. She helped us during our previous three births and we felt comfortable having her there in this capacity. At 7:15 A.M., I had a very long and strong contraction while Rick was taking a shower, and suddenly my water broke. This was the first time it happened during the early part of my labor; in the past it broke in transition.

My contractions gradually became stronger and closer together and I settled on the couch with the heating pad on my lower back. The heat, plus Rick pushing hard on my lower back during each contraction felt so good. During the contractions, my eyes would focus on the Sacred Heart of Jesus, whose picture we have hanging over our family shrine. This brought tremendous consolation. I knew he was there with us, protecting us, as we brought a child of His into the world.

After awhile it just seemed like I couldn't get in a comfortable position. Rick was holding me and helping me through each contraction. When it started to become difficult, Regina boiled water and brought it to Rick so he could apply hot towels on my abdomen, inner thighs and perineum. This was so helpful; the hot towels seemed to

---

The Autumn of Love: As a result of tending the garden during the summer, we get to harvest the results of our hard work. Fall has come. It is golden time—rich and fulfilling. We experience a more mature love that accepts and understands our partner's imperfections as well as our own. It is a time of thanksgiving and sharing. Having worked hard during summer we can relax and enjoy the love we have created. —John Gray

absorb much of the pain. I became so hot and sweaty during transition that all I wanted was to put cold cloths over my face and suck on raspberry leaf tea ice cubes.

Rick checked to see if he could tell how far dilated I was. He said he could feel the baby's head, but was not sure if he could feel any cervix around it. It was uncomfortable for me, but he kept trying. After a few very strong contractions, I began to feel better by pushing gently when the pain was at its greatest.

It wasn't long before I could feel the baby descending and Rick saying, "The baby's coming. The head is almost out." Another push and Timothy was born. Rick yelled, "Get the cord!" when he saw that it was wrapped tightly around his neck twice. I knew this was common and said, "It's okay. We'll just unwrap it." As soon as we unwrapped the cord, Timothy cried and we all relaxed. Rick said, "It's a boy!" and I took him and laid back on the couch with him. We had hoped that Conrad, our five year old and only son until now, would have a baby brother.

His breathing was somewhat raspy, so I suctioned his mouth gently with the bulb syringe. I put him to my breast and he began to nurse. His face, hands and feet were blue at birth, but he pinked right up. Regina cut the cord after ten minutes when it stopped pulsating and was very limp. Rick milked enough blood out of it for the blood tube to check the baby's blood type since we were unsure whether or not I should get Rhogam if the baby's blood was Rh positive.

The placenta came out thirty minutes later and Rick buried it in our garden. After Timmy stopped nursing, Regina got me a basin of warm water to put him in for a few minutes. I wanted to do this at the other births, but never seemed to have the opportunity. Although I was not bleeding, I took some Shepherd's Purse to clamp down the uterus. I had not torn at all. Rick said that as the baby emerged, the skin stretched around him as it was supposed to.

Timothy did turn out to be Rh positive, but we decided that I would not receive the Rhogam injection. When researching whether to take the Rhogam shot or not, I found that the mother's and baby's blood is most likely to mix in a hospital setting, where they pull on the cord to yank out the placenta or when the cord is clamped early, leading to a back-up of fetal blood into the mother's circulation. This is not normal conduct in a homebirth, so we decided to leave these matters into God's hands.

I feel that it is important to add that following the birth, it means so much to have your husband stay with you for as long as possible just to be together to share your feelings about the event. The day after Timothy's birth, Rick drove 200 miles each way to bring my mom to see the new baby. I was very happy to see my mom and have her help, but feel that we missed out on something very important that day—the quiet intimacy—that we have been unable to recapture ever since.

I cannot accurately describe the satisfaction I feel from this birth, and the increased love I have for God who has directed us towards this way (His way) of birthing, and for my husband who has never left my side, and supported me through it all. I also give thanks to our daughter Regina, who totally respected our privacy, yet was always there when she was needed. I hope it has been helpful to her as she enters adulthood with the right attitudes about marriage, love, family and birthing. This birth has given Rick and I an increased mutual appreciation for each other and our family. For us, this was not as much a sexual as it was an emotionally intimate experience. If we are blessed with more children, we will certainly birth them in the same way.

I am 44 and Tim is now four years old. During the past four years, I have had four early, but upsetting miscarriages. When I became pregnant again, I was fully expecting another. I was relieved when I felt the baby's first movements.

I did not see a doctor during this pregnancy at all. With each pregnancy, we took more responsibility and were much happier for it. In the past it seemed like any "assistance" always turned out to be negative for us. I only had one blood test for Rh antibodies in the early months and stopped taking Rhogam after my fifth baby. The test was negative so I didn't think anymore about it. I kept weekly tabs on my blood pressure and always tried to eat well, especially lots of protein. I also took supplements and herbs.

At 5:00 A.M. on September 18, I woke up and realized I was in early labor. Our oldest daughters left for work while the others left for school. My friend Debbie offered to watch Tim. Once labor really got underway, I felt most comfortable sitting up straight and breathing deeply. When the labor became intense and difficult, I moved from the rocker to the birthing stool that Rick made. Our supplies were on a small table close by.

Rick tried twice during labor to see how far dilated I was, but said he wasn't sure what he was feeling. Then I began to shake and he knew I was in transition. I got to the point where I felt I had to push, so I did. After a few of these contractions, I felt the baby's head move down into the birth canal. It was 4:50 P.M. and I was very excited to finally be making progress. In two more contractions, Rick said, "The head is out," and with the next one I pushed out the rest of our baby. He caught our little girl—thanks be to God! What a relief! She was slightly blue, but cried right away. She nursed well, a little bit at a time. This moment right after birth is the greatest feeling of a lifetime! I will always relish it. Regina and Gretchen got back home about 20 minutes before her birth. They heard the "strange noises" I was making even before they came into the house. We spent about an hour just enjoying our new little one and waiting for the placenta. We didn't cut the cord until after the placenta was out. I took some Shepherd's Purse tincture to be sure I wouldn't bleed excessively.

We did have one scare about 1-1/2 hours after her birth. She turned blue and seemed to have stopped breathing. Rick noticed it first and was very scared. I immediately put her over my thigh and stroked her back a little vigorously and right away she began to have little cries again. I continued stroking her and talking to her to be sure she wouldn't stop again. There was never a problem after that. I felt sure that since she began crying and breathing fine right after the birth, and didn't seem to be congested at all, she would breathe again without much coaxing.

We named our little girl Pauline Catherine after two favorite aunts, and also after the sister of St. Therese of Lisieux, whom she chose to take the place of her mother after she died. Pauline weighed 8 lbs. 12 oz. at birth and I only had one small tear. I think I had torn there during a previous birth. Rick did use olive oil to massage my perineum when birth was imminent, but perhaps if we had used it earlier, I wouldn't have torn at all.

All our children were thrilled to come home and meet little Pauline—they all just love her to pieces. Rick and I are completely enraptured with her. We are, above all, deeply grateful to God for giving us this beautiful baby (at our age and after so many miscarriages) and the wisdom, knowledge, strength and trust to birth our baby alone at home in accordance with His designs for normal childbirth. Deo Gratias!

23

Continuity, Peace and Harmony

Jesse and Kirstina Wimberley
Southbend, NC
Generations to Come

Kirstina believes that an unassisted birth is as important for the husband to experience as the wife. Involving your lover in childbirth will profoundly affect his life. Cody and Sophia Wimberley had the privilege of being members of their family's fourth generation to be born in the same house. A more lengthy discussion of the Wimberley's birth story appears in Chapter 9.

This is not luck, but decision-making, responsibility, self-confidence and educating oneself in the process of birthing, the anatomy and physiology of birthing. I had three homebirths and this was Jesse's first child, Cody. Our second child, Sophia was also an unassisted homebirth. I have two other children from a prior marriage. My first child, Sunflower ("Sunny"), was with a midwife, but after a 21-hour labor, the midwife induced me with castor oil and the baby wasn't ready to come out; it wasn't time yet. I ended up in the hospital.

We decided then that we didn't want to have another assisted birth and wanted to do it ourselves. Kai Indigo was born at home after a three-hour labor in the waterbag with me leaning against his dad with just his sister there and a friend. Cody was my third birth and Sophia was the fourth.

Details of Cody's birth: He had the cord wrapped around his neck and Jesse just removed that instinctively. He probably forgot everything he read, but just acted out of instinct. He was also born with meconium on him and had no water. He must have been dehydrated and the waterbag never broke. All of the four children had meconium on them. It's not such a scary scene. It's way overestimated. We waited for the placenta to come out and Sunny and Kai cut the cord after about ten minutes and we had clamps we put on it. Jesse, Sunflower and Kai buried the placenta under a fig tree.

None of the births went according to the medical textbook description as far as a bloody show first, waterbags breaking, things like that. We had to suction Cody's nose with a small bulb syringe because he had swallowed some meconium.

Scott and Charity Gregson
Bremerton, WA
Waterbirth

The Gregson's have six children. The first two were born in the hospital and the last four were DIY births. Their first and fourth DIYs are described here with a few brief comments on what they did differently during the second and third DIY.

Jason Andrew (11/9/91): At the time of our third pregnancy, we had not heard of anyone birthing their baby without a doctor or midwife's assistance. Of course, almost everybody has heard of the native women who would go off into the woods and come back a short time later with their newborn baby. But in America, it's just not done that way anymore, or so the medical community would have you think.

We had had two rather easy and uneventful, natural hospital births (except for a mild case of shoulder dystocia, which the doctor had little trouble releasing). Roy, our firstborn, weighed 9 lbs., 12 oz. in December, 1988. At the birth of our daughter Sally on June 3, 1990, the doctor arrived just in time to put his gloves on, sit down and catch the baby. After a move across the country and a new job, in early 1991 we found ourselves expecting a third baby, but now we had no medical insurance. After consulting with a couple of local midwives, we knew we could not afford to go that way either.

One day, about three months into the pregnancy, my husband Scott asked me why we couldn't just have the baby at home ourselves. I had already considered this option, but did not say anything because I thought he would never go for it. We talked about it, considered that my labors and births were very easy, and decided that we didn't need medical assistance for such a natural process as childbirth. We purchased a blood pressure cuff and a stethoscope so we could keep a prenatal record. We wanted to have this as proof that we had prenatal care, not knowing how the legal system would react if anything tragic happened to either me or the baby.

Through a local midwife, I found out about a birthing supply company in Oregon and sent away for their catalog. We also purchased *William's Obstetrics*, a textbook used in medical school. We read up on all the different complications and how to handle them. The chances of any of these complications happening was unlikely. I decided that someday I wanted to become a midwife and I read every pregnancy and birth book I could get my hands on. I discovered what a natural process birth is and never felt any anxiety at all about our future unassisted birth.

I told anyone who asked that we were planning a DIY birth, but after some bad reactions from a few people, I was more cautious of who I told. I even found out after the birth that one person had planned to call 911 and have an ambulance sent to our house when I was in labor. Needless to say, I was glad he did not hear anything until after the baby was born.

In September, we ordered supplies. Surgical gloves would be used by Scott to reduce the possibility of the baby or me getting an infection. A bulb syringe would be on hand for clearing the baby's air passages. We ordered plastic cord clamps, absorbent underpads, a large plastic bag for covering our mattress, an antibacterial handwash, sanitary pads and briefs and a few other things.

My due date passed with no sign of the baby, but my Braxton Hicks contractions became more frequent. On the evening of November 8, I noticed some bloody show. My husband checked, but there was no real change from the time before. I called my mother, who would be taking my children to her house during the birth, to let her know of the new development. I told her it may still be days away, but I just wanted her to be prepared. I also called my sister and friend who would be coming to take photos of the birth and to help out.

We went to bed and I was awakened by a contraction at 2:30 A.M. Ten minutes later, I had another contraction. During the next 45 minutes, they got stronger and closer together. I woke up Scott and he checked my cervix again. We put the plastic mattress cover over our mattress and made the bed. It was just after 3:30 A.M. and I decided to pass the time folding laundry. My husband thought I was crazy, but I figured, "Why not? I can't sleep anyway." By 5 A.M. I knew it was time to call everyone. The contractions were averaging six minutes apart and were getting very uncomfortable. I was so glad I would be staying in my own house rather than traveling to the hospital.

I called my friend Marla and we got the kids dressed and fed. My mom was marveling that I was so intent on getting the laundry done. My husband told me to forget about the laundry and that he would do it later. When my mom and kids left at 6:30 A.M., Scott checked my cervix and it was five centimeters dilated. My contractions were about four minutes apart and I had fleeting thoughts of, "Will I really be able to do this at home?" The next couple of hours were a blur of one contraction after another.

Scott set out the birthing supplies. At 8:45 A.M., Scott thought that I was all the way open, but there was a large bubble of the bag of water bulging in front of the head. I said we should try to break it so it would be easier to push the baby out. We knew by feeling from the outside that this was another large baby. After about twenty minutes of trying to break the water bag with sterile items, it finally popped with a gush. I felt so much relief. I got up on our bed and the urge to push took over. Alice started snapping pictures. After just three pushes, Scott caught Jason at 9:28 A.M. He weighed 9 lbs. 2 oz. We got a couple of good pictures of Scott catching him. I had no vaginal tears at all and after Scott clamped the cord, Alice cut it. The placenta came soon with no problems. I took a shower within 45 minutes and felt wonderful.

WOW! What an experience! That was one of the major highs of my life. I felt like I was "floating" for weeks afterward. We felt thankful to have been blessed with such an easy birth in our own home and I knew that I didn't ever want to birth in a hospital again. I scheduled an appointment with the County Health Department's Well Baby Clinic. Our son was examined that first week and he was pronounced a very healthy baby. I had been a little nervous about how the nurse would react to the circumstances of his birth, but she turned out to have no negative remarks at all. We filed for a birth certificate with the county registrar within a month, which was a very easy process to fulfill.

Johnathan David (3/27/93): Labor during my fourth pregnancy and second DIY birth was also very long and drawn out. Although my cervix was ready to deliver a baby, it seemed as if the baby was taking its time. We decided to try to get the head to engage by pressing down on the top of the fundus during a contraction and holding it there. After doing this for a few contractions, we did get the head lower down. Scott checked the heart rate and it was still good. We held the head in place for about four contractions to make sure it wouldn't go back up. The baby's heart rate remained strong throughout the entire procedure.

Our birthing supplies were set in the kitchen and we used a homemade birthing stool so that I could deliver upright with the help of gravity. Although I felt no urge to push, my husband told me to push to see what would happen. Soon afterwards, he was shouting, "Stop pushing! Stop pushing! Breathe, breathe." I couldn't stop; the baby was coming out on its own. Suddenly, the baby shot out, along with the amniotic fluid from the sac breaking. Scott almost dropped the baby because it was coming out so fast. He was unprepared for such a fast delivery.

After a visit with the Well Child Clinic, they determined that my son had a club foot; his right foot and ankle had a deformity. The muscles had grown so that the foot would not flex. If not corrected early enough, the bones may harden in the wrong position. We were referred to the Children's Hospital in Seattle and his foot was corrected using casting and a brace. Others have to have surgery to correct the problem. We filed for his birth certificate and SSN and thanked God for another blessing born into his father's hands.

<u>Nathan Scott (6/16/95)</u>: One thing I did differently during this labor was to drink castor oil to make myself go into labor. All it did was make me sick. During the pushing phase, the baby came slowly. I was concerned because our first baby had shoulder dystocia and I remember the doctor and nurse pushing on my belly to help get him out. We attempted this and decided I should try to lay down on the floor. As I stood up with the baby's head hanging out of me, I felt something shift inside of me and decided to push again. Out came our 10 lb. 8 oz. son without any tearing of my body. Before he was two weeks old, we took him to the Well Child Clinic. They didn't like it that we refused a PKU test and immunizations, but we feel that they are unnecessary. We applied for his birth certificate and SSN. Words cannot describe the euphoria we felt.

<u>Abigail Suzanne (11/04/96)</u>: During my studies to become a midwife, I viewed a video of a waterbirth and decided that our next baby would be born in the water. At first, my husband was apprehensive about having a waterbirth, but as his questions were answered ("What if the baby inhales water as

it is being born? How do you know how much blood the mother loses?"), we began searching for a tub. We discovered a business that rented tubs for waterbirth at a cost of $150.00. While this is definitely worth it, we could not afford it and began looking for children's pools. Since it was at the end of the season, I could not find a pool and asked the owner of the store if we could make some type of arrangement about renting the tub. She had a tub in storage that she would rent for $50.00 and agreed to sell it to me if I liked it!

Once again, I went past my due date and was well into my 43rd week of pregnancy. The baby's head was not engaged and by Nov. 2, I tried to stimulate some contractions by twisting my nipples. After only five minutes, I started having contractions 7-8 minutes apart. This was after not having any contractions during the whole day. After an hour, I decided to go to bed, hoping the contractions would continue. They wouldn't and I asked a childbirth educator friend for some advice. She said to continue the nipple stimulation until I was five centimeters dilated and contractions were well established.

The nipple stimulation directly effected my labor. If I quit, labor would come to a halt and if I continued, I felt as if we were making progress. After five hours of pumping, disinfecting and filling the inflatable tub with hot tap water, we were ready for our new baby. I continued nipple stimulation and we applied fundal pressure to try to get the baby to drop. I stepped into the tub and I felt totally weightless. It was so easy to move around in different positions. I was so exhausted and tried to lay down, but labor was finally progressing. I got back into the water at 1:30 A.M. I was amazed at how much easier the contractions were to handle while I was immersed in the soothing water.

I get real vocal when I go through transition and when Scott heard the loud moans coming from the kitchen, he knew it was time to check on my progress. It was now about 2:20 A.M. and I knew this baby would be born within two hours. When Scott checked my cervix, it took him a while to say that I had made no progress. I was so discouraged and as he continued checking, he thought I was completed dilated. It was difficult to tell in the water. We forgot to lay out the birth supplies and I was ready to push the baby out within seconds. When I began to push, I noticed that it was much harder to push under water than with my five dry births. The books on waterbirth had mentioned this, but now I was experiencing it.

After two pushes, the baby's head was out, and I decided it might be easier to push if I was on my hands and knees. Because we didn't have the tub full, the baby's face was above the surface of the water. We had planned to birth the baby completely underwater, but the books advised against keeping the baby's face under the water after it had been exposed to the air. The cold air might trigger the breathing reflex. After one more push, out slid the baby into Daddy's hands at 2:34 A.M. The first thing Scott said was, "It's a girl!" I was so excited. Linda and Alice were screaming and cheering because they knew I wanted another girl. We did not take her to the Well Child Clinic as we had with the other children. We did register her birth and get her SSN though.

I am definitely a waterbirth proponent now. The labor was by far the easiest one I've had. We decided to purchase the tub so it will be available if I should ever need it again. She is working out a special payment plan for us. Also, I will rent it out to others in my community who want to experience the joy of waterbirthing. I recommend waterbirthing to anyone.

24

Breech Twins

Peter and Judie
Ewing, NJ
Promised Blessings

Peter and Judie decided that they were not going to allow medical professionals "ownership" of their pregnancy. They refused to submit to a system that performs C-sections on breech twins simply because of fear or custom. Peter and Judie decided on a courageous approach to birth rather than a cowardly medical delivery. Luke and Dylan were born on April 29, 1996.

My third pregnancy was a long awaited answer to prayer. We had already had two sons who were five and seven and growing like weeds in a garden. We all ached to hold a brand new baby in our arms. We prayed often and the next thing we knew, I conceived.

In the beginning, I had voiced my feelings about a homebirth and wanted to see one of my favorite midwives, who had worked at a birthing center where I once sought prenatal care. She now had her own midwifery center and was only one mile from my home. I thought this would be perfect until I discovered that our insurance would not accept her for coverage. I was upset and allowed myself to believe that the only answer I had was to return to the birthing center where I was cared for with my two older sons.

I hated the idea of seeing this one particular midwife with whom I did not see eye-to-eye. It just so happened that on my very first day of prenatal care she was the one who greeted and examined me. During the third month of my pregnancy we discovered we were expecting twins. We were so excited, especially the boys. They told everyone that they each had their own baby to care for and love. During the sixth month I began to have complications with spotting. I had to go into the hospital for IV feedings and then realized that I had not consumed enough liquids for twins. I began drinking a gallon of fluids each day and was constantly using the bathroom.

I was exhausted, but my spirits were high. Then we were told that both babies had turned and were breech. We were informed that they would probably arrive early, as most twins do. I became irritated with the birthing center visits, along with hospital visits, words that were not encouraging, and the two types of ultrasound visits they told me were necessary. I was tired of all this nonsense and I especially disliked their flippant attitude that "after 35 weeks, it's okay to schedule a date for a cesarean section." I still yearned for a homebirth and jokingly told Peter this is what we were going to have.

I searched the local libraries for books on different types of births and then one day in the mail I received a magazine that had an ad with free information on homebirthing. I wrote and promptly received a list of books on homebirths. I ordered the books and read to my heart's content. Peter said that he had never seen me so interested in reading and sharing every detail of what I had read. He was amazed and listened as I poured out my heart about my desire to have a homebirth. We prayed about it and had the peace of mind that this was what God wanted us to do.

On April 1, 1996 I called the birthing center and told them what we had decided. We would no longer be in need of their services. The center did not like what we had decided and sent us a letter warning us of the dangers and allowing us so many hours to change our minds and resume care with them. We did not allow their scare tactics to rob us of our promised blessings, and so we continued with our plans.

It's funny how I began having impulsive labor pains just hours after informing the birthing center of our plans. My due date was 28 days away and we prayed that the babies would not come early. The false labor continued each day, with several contractions a day. Peter said we should pray about this and so we did. I felt my body widening and preparing for birth with each contraction. On Sunday, April 28, Peter asked, "Will I have to go to work tomorrow?" That was his way of saying how he hated to see the weekends come to an end. I just smiled. We all went to bed as usual, except Peter and I had a little intimate time before falling asleep. At about 3:52 A.M., I had a sudden urge to urinate and it was strange that I tried to roll over on my belly. Of course this was impossible, so I backed to the foot end of our bed, grabbed the bed rail and backed down to the floor. I made it to the bathroom and I found that I could not stop urinating. There was a continual dripping and then it dawned on me; my amniotic sac had broken!

I was excited, but I could not lift myself up from the toilet as I feared soaking the floor. I sat there for about fifteen minutes waiting for the dripping to stop. It didn't, so I put a washcloth between my legs, walked into our bedroom, turned the lights on and told Peter to wake up and start preparing for the babies. I recall him staring at me like, "You do not look like you're in labor," and I am sure I did not because I felt no pain. I walked back into our bathroom to take a shower and felt something like a bubble extending from my vagina. Peter was standing in the bathroom doorway.

I excitedly said, "Pete! Here come the babies!" The bubble burst and the widening pressure was hard and breathtaking. The floor was now soaked and Peter wanted me to hurry to the bedroom, but I still wanted my shower. While showering, I felt everything within me bearing down. I called out to Jesus, thanking him for his promises and I heard Peter talking to Jesus on the outside of the shower curtain. He helped me out, dried me and rushed me into the bedroom. I had no desire to get onto the bed.

I stood at our computer desk and told Peter to prepare for the babies as they were coming down at that very moment. I asked Peter to read aloud the Bible verses we had hung up all around our bedroom. He read several while standing next to me, holding me. Then he knelt down and saw baby #1 coming out. He tried to put on plastic gloves, which was a funny sight to behold. He ripped the things up and threw them aside to catch his first son, who was coming forth, buttock breech. Peter was quiet for a few seconds and then he calmly asked me to push. I told him that I didn't have the urge to push. A second later, this baby who was stuck from the rib cage up came sliding out on his own. Following him was his sac. Peter quickly reached for a towel and cleaned Dylan's nose and wrapped him.

I told him to hurry because baby #2 was coming out. I stood at the computer desk bearing down, asking Peter to hurry as I did not want this child to land on the floor. Peter crawled over to me with Dylan in his left arm and seeing our second son arriving still in his sac. Peter peeled the sac away and saw another buttock breech coming down. He held onto his little rear-end and guided him to safety. Luke's cord was attached to me so Peter told me to walk backwards to our bed, where I sat and held Dylan, while Peter cleaned Luke's nose and wrapped him. The babies were born three minutes apart, 4:54 A.M. and 4:57 A.M. on April 29, 1996, their due date.

My total time of discomfort was about 35 minutes, with 25 minutes of waiting for the leakage to stop. I pushed Luke's placenta into a bucket about ten minutes after Luke was born. I sat up in bed and Peter and I admired our two new arrivals. We heard a gentle knock at the bedroom door and it was our seven year-old son, Jared. He said he heard a baby's cry and wanted to see. He held Luke, who resembled him when he was a newborn baby. He was in love with his new siblings. Hours later, six year-old Adanh woke up and rushed into our bedroom. He was excited and happy and shouted, "My babies are here!" Dylan and Luke are a definite reminder of God's wonderful promises to his children. We are still amazed, and give thanks everyday.

AFTERWORD

We desire success and fulfillment in our lives. Success in life is often contingent upon how much effort we put forth. The more responsibility we take and the more knowledge we have entering into a situation (like birth), the more prepared we will be for problems. We can react to situations which require quick thinking.

Unassisted homebirth is not only an act of love, but a gift of love. Women who decide upon unassisted birth tap into resources of faith and wisdom, while husbands who have not given much thought to birth are given the gift of involvement by their wives. Couples who set goals for birth and commit themselves to an unassisted homebirth have a great chance of emerging from a rite of passage not only with satisfaction, but a stronger bond.

If you are thinking, "Great. Now that I read this book, I *have* to have an unassisted birth, but where do I start? Can I do this? Can we really do it?"

Begin by asking "what if" questions. "What will I do if the cord is wrapped around the baby's neck?" Go find an answer you are satisfied with and then ask another question and find another answer. Before you know it, you will have done a lot of research, built up confidence and eliminated fears. It is only natural that you will encounter doubt and fear. I would be suspicious of someone who was 100% confident and had no questions or concerns. Talk to others who have had unassisted homebirths. They are out there, but you may have to work hard to find them.

A key thought I would like to leave with you is that anyone can have an unassisted homebirth—it doesn't take an expert to bring forth a child. So many people will try to convince you that you are incapable of birthing your own child, and that you must be an expert. When we can learn to trust the process of birth, we will enjoy our births much more.

Trust, pray, exercise, eat right, visualize, detach yourself from negative and nosy people. Talk with your spouse about the pregnancy and birth. Order as few or as many birth supplies as you think you will need. And then you will have an awesome story to tell and lots of love to share, because unassisted homebirth is truly an act of love.

Wishing you love and happiness on your parenting journey, beginning with your birth experience,

Lynn M. Griesemer

Request for personal stories

I am continuing to study unassisted homebirth and am interested in receiving personal stories. If you would like to share your birth story, send it to me at Terra Publishing, P.O. Box 80514, Charleston, SC 29416-0514.

email: greeze@juno.com

website: http://ourworld.compuserve.com/homepages/bgriesemer.

Please indicate whether I may have permission to publicly share or reprint your story.

APPENDIX A
Final Thoughts

As you have seen, profound changes have taken place in the lives of couples who have had DIY homebirths. Many of the couples wanted to share comments and resources that helped them prepare for the big event .

Did you have the birth videotaped, photographed, audiotaped? What were the pros and cons in your experience?

We got photographs after the birth because there was no one there to take them. I feel that this was a major draw-back because I was looking forward to having photos of the birth.

No. We took a few photos afterwards. I have a personal preference to have no visual record of the birth. It would be too weird to see myself labor.

With our first DIY, no, since it was too hectic. We had an assistant to take pictures at our next DIY.

No, although I attended a birth that was videotaped. We were happy just to have photos immediately after birth.

No. It would have been nice to record the blessed event. On the other hand, that would mean my husband would be concentrating on equipment rather than me. Being recorded alters and inhibits the mood.

No, we feel this would be intrusive and to relive it again by audio or video would lessen the "specialness" of it. We have photographed other births, but our thinking has changed.

No, we originally wanted it videotaped and it would be nice to have that, but the possible negative vibes of someone else being there was not worth it.

Our first two DIYs were photographed and last two were videotaped. We wanted photos of the last two, but they were forgotten in the excitement of the moment. I'm very glad for the videotape. Next time we will have someone present whose only job is to take photos of the whole thing.

No. We feel that the birth of our children is as intimate and private as conception.

Unfortunately, no one was able to videotape my homebirth. I had my sister lined up to do the job but she was unable to make it.

If you have had a DIY homebirth and would not do it again, why?

Most of the couples would opt for a DIY again. All of the women were confident and comfortable without anyone else present. Those whose husbands were apprehensive would welcome a skilled childbirth supporter or friend.

One of the unplanned DIY mother's believes that her husband would prefer an attendant since he was nervous. The other couple had a DIY birth with their next child.

Any other suggestions or comments?

My two DIY births are the greatest blessings of our lives. Thank you for doing all this research to help others make the same wonderful decision—to have great births which affect our children forever.

My suggestion is to inform people how safe homebirth really is. A lot of people thought we were very irresponsible for having a homebirth. I think they are irresponsible for trusting their doctors so fully.

In another question, you asked if I felt more connected to my DIY child. It's not that I love my new baby more than my first (hospital-born), but with my first, I had this terrible paranoia that someone at the hospital had switched babies. There was a belligerent labor nurse that I somehow didn't trust, and after they took my baby away to bathe and measure, she came back in the room with a different wrist tag saying that the old ones were misspelled. When I got Celeste back after almost three hours, she looked different!

It sounds crazy, but until I later compared the pictures of her when she was first born to the baby in my arms, I was afraid she wasn't mine. I've had to live with the guilt, shame and anger ever since. With Corinne, there was never that awful, paranoid doubt. No one took my baby away! No strange labor nurses or unwelcome guests in my home!

One suggestion would be to emphasize the importance of registering the homebirth with the county's vital records' office. It is a very simple procedure, and it is important that all homebirths be accounted for, as there are studies done to show the safety of homebirths.

Whenever you feel uncomfortable or uneasy with your medical care, don't sit there like a frog on a log. Don't let the so called medical professionals make you feel as though you know nothing. Don't allow yourself to be put onto a conveyor belt and pushed along at their convenience. Speak up and let your OB/Gyn know exactly how you feel, and if they can't help you then it is best for you to leave their establishment.

What topics should be written about or researched regarding homebirths?

I think it's important to know how different couples handle problems that occur during birth to give others ideas about this. It seems most people are adverse to DIY birth because "something may go wrong." Those people should know that those things are usually minor and easily dealt with.

A lot of people think homebirth is nearly impossible and that it is difficult to find a midwife to attend your birth at home. Homebirth is a lot easier than they think.

The psychological aspects for women after a homebirth. The renewed sense of self and empowerment. The ability to trust and listen to our inner voice / intuition and the courage to follow it.

How breech babies can be safely delivered without cesarean delivery.

I would be interested in reading about the attitude of different doctors and midwives regarding DIY homebirths. Also, whether parents have been prosecuted for the death or maiming of a child or any other aspect pertaining to DIY birth.

What are some resources that helped you prepare for the birth?
(not listed in the bibliography)

The Bible
Dr. Christopher's Herbal Class and Books, correspondence school. 1-800-372-8255.
A Woman's View of Her Body, The Federation of Feminist Women's Health Centers, 1981, Touchtone.
Heart and Hands: A Guide to Midwifery by Elizabeth Davis. 1981, Bantam Books, NY, NY.
Primal Connection by Elizabeth Nobel, Simon & Schuster, NY.
Pregnancy, Childbirth and Newborn. Peggy Simkin, Janet Whalley, and Ann Keppler. 1991, Meadowbrook Press, Simon & Schuster, 1230 Avenue of the Americas, NY, NY.

William's Obstetrics
Childbirth: God's Way by Brenda Willis.
Complications of Labor and Delivery by Valerie Hobbs. 1982.
Survival into the 21st Century by Victoras Kulvinskas. 1975, 21ˢᵗ Century Publications, P.O.Box 64, Woodstock Valley, CT 06282.
Wise Woman Herbal for the Childbearing Year by Susun S. Weed. 1986. Ashtree Publishing Co., Woodstock, NY.
What Every Pregnant Woman Should Know: The Truth about diet and drugs during Pregnancy. Brewer, Tom M.D., and Gail Sforza.1977, Random House, NY.
Waterbirth by Janet Balaskas
The Waterbirth Handbook by Dr. Lichy and Eileen Herzberg.
Women Giving Birth by Lindburg and Smulders.
Children at Birth
Safe Alternatives in Childbirth
American Academy of Husband-Coached Childbirth
Local Homebirth Association meetings with other couples.
The Joy of Natural Childbirth, 5th ed. by Helen Wessel. 1994, Bookmates International, Inc., Fresno, CA.
Silent Knife: Cesarean Prevention and Vaginal Birth after Cesarean by Nancy Wainer Cohen and Lois J. Estner. 1983, Bergin & Garvey Publishers, Westport, CT.
Primal Mothering in a Modern World by Hygeia Halfmoon. P.O. Box 1275, Pahoa, HI 96778, 1-800-788-1740.
I Can Do This! Excerpts from an Expectant Woman. by Hygeia Halfmoon. P.O.Box 1275, Pahoa, HI 96778.

APPENDIX B
Additional Resources

Newsletters / Magazines

1. *The New Nativity II.* Newsletter for Do-it-Yourself Home-birth couples. Edited by Valarie Nordstrom. 4820 69th Ave. No., Brooklyn Center, MN 55429-1673. Published four times a year, $10.00 subscription.
2. *The Compleat Mother: The Magazine of Pregnancy, Birth and Breastfeeding.* P.O. Box 209, Minot, ND 58702. Published four times a year, $12.00 subscription.

Catalogs/Birth Supplies

Cascade Healthcare Products, Inc. (Birth & Life Bookstore; Moonflower Birthing Supply), 141 Commercial St. NE, Salem, OR 97301. (503) 371-4445.
Yalad Birthing Supply, P. O. Box 8111, Canton, OH 44711-8111. (216) 499-0679.
Spirt-Led Childbirth. P.O. Box 1225, Oakhurst, CA 93644. 1-888-683-2678

Fertility Awareness

Balsam, Charles & Elizabeth. *Family Planning: A Guide for Exploring the Issues,* 3rd ed. 1994, Liguori Publications,

Liguori, MO.

Billings, John. *The Ovulation Method.* 1972, Borromeo Guild, Los Angeles, CA.

Kippley, John & Sheila. *The Art of Natural Family Planning,* 3rd ed. 1984, Couple to Couple League International, Inc., Cincinnati, OH.

Kippley, Sheila. *Breastfeeding & Natural Child Spacing: How "Ecological Breastfeeding Spaces Babies.* 2nd ed., 1989, Couple to Couple League International, Inc., Cincinnati, OH.

Nofziger, Margaret. *A Cooperative Method of Natural Birth Control.* 1976, The Book Publishing Co., Summertown, TN.

Weschler, Toni. *Taking Charge of Your Fertility: The Definitive Guide to Natural Birth Control & Pregnancy Achievement.* 1995, Harper Collins Pub., NY, NY.

Winstein, Merryl. *Your Fertility Signals: Using them to Achieve or Avoid Pregnancy, Naturally.* 1989, Smooth Stone Press, St. Louis, MO.

APPENDIX C
The Questionnaire

TO: Home Birth Couple   10/28/96

Thank you for your inquiry about the homebirth book project I am working on. I would like to publish a book at the end of 1997 to benefit couples considering homebirths and as a resource for those who support homebirths. I have decided that the book will focus on unassisted homebirths / "Do-it-Yourself" (DIY) homebirths which occured after 1/1/90. If you know of anyone else who has had a DIY homebirth after 1/1/90 and would like to participate, feel free to provide them copies of this questionnaire. I want to show that a variety of people choose to have unassisted homebirths. My goal is to incorporate 20 personal homebirth stories which will consist of about half of the book. I would be satisfied with 10 solid stories though. Return your story to me at the above address.

As for why I'm doing this project: I have no special qualifications, just a strong desire to share information with others. I'm a mother of five and recently experienced our first homebirth (DIY) after four hospital deliveries. I feel compelled to speak out about many issues surrounding homebirths.

The book will be mostly a presentation of unassisted homebirth as it relates to psychological growth and development—of the couple, the woman, the man. Some issues I will focus on include: self-actualization; men's experience of the birth; midwives role in the birth process; secrets doctors will never tell you. It won't be a how-to book, but more of an experiential book. Some people consider DIY homebirthers as one extreme of the childbirth spectrum. I would also like to present some stories of the minority among DIY homebirthers—such as a water birth or first baby a DIY.

Every question I ask is relevant to my theses / hypotheses and actual writing of the book. If you would rather not answer some of the questions or feel that they are intrusive, feel free to leave them blank. Please read through the entire questionnaire before you begin and call me if you need clarification. You may write your responses on the questionnaire and/ or use additional pages of your own. As long as you address each issue, by all means, use your own style. I know better than to try to put restrictions on homebirthers!

Information you provide will be kept confidential and used for this project only. I know that it may be very difficult to put your experiences into words, but try the best you can so that we can communicate the wonderful experience of unassisted homebirths with others. Thank you for your participation and I will be in touch with you at a later date.

Sincerely,

Lynn M. Griesemer

UNASSISTED HOMEBIRTH QUESTIONNAIRE

<u>PART I. BACKGROUND INFORMATION</u>

1. Couple's name, address, phone number, Email, fax:
2. Has the birth story you are submitting to me ever been published?_____If yes, where?
3. Where / How did you find out about this research I am doing?
4. I will not print addresses or phone numbers in the final product. Do you have any objection to me listing your full

names, city and state?_____ If yes, how would you prefer me to identify you?

5. Indicate names of your children, birthdate, place born (hospital, birthing center, home or specify other), "delivered" by who, who watched the birth/was present at the birth.

Child's name	Birthdate	Place Born	Delivered by who	Who witnessed the birth
				(Ob/Gyn; midwife; husband, etc.)

6. Father's highest educational degree:
   Mother's highest educational degree:
   Father's job / profession:
   Mother's current job / profession:
   Mother's job / profession before children:
7. Briefly state why you had a DIY homebirth:
8. I have noticed that many homebirthers are very committed to childbearing, childrearing and are very family oriented. Many homebirthers embrace a "natural" lifestyle. What other family lifestyle practices do you feel strongly about or have incorporated into your life? (examples: extended breastfeeding; family bed; cloth diapers; homeschoolers; vegetarian/ nutrition conscious/ natural hygiene; work from the home; no immunizations; no circumcisions; believe in homeopathic remedies rather than traditional medical practices; fertility awareness / natural family planning method of birth control; athletic family; involved in community or church activities; etc.) Is there anything your family does together daily (such as always try to eat the dinner meal, pray together, some family habit that brings you closer):

PART II. PREGNANCY QUESTIONS

1. What type of prenatal care did you receive, your level of exercise, how you felt physically throughout the pregnancy, whether you believe you had good nutrition habits, any special problems throughout the pregnancy. I want to know went well for you too.
2. How was your frame of mind regarding fear, anxiety, tension during the pregnancy?

How did you cope with it or prepare yourself to deal with fear, if you experienced it?

Mother:

Father:

3. I want to devote a chapter of the book to "Secrets your doctor will never tell you." What can you share about pregnancy and delivery that we don't often find written about? An example would be: Drink raspberry leaf tea throughout pregnancy to tone up your uterus and during delivery, be patient about expelling the placenta to prevent hemorrhaging.

PART III. DELIVERY / BIRTH QUESTIONS

1. What are some techniques, strategies or practices you can share that helped you have a smooth delivery?

2. What birth supplies did you have ready?

3. Did you do any internal exams to check dilation or effacement?

4. Did you have an emergency / back-up plans? If yes, briefly explain.

5. Did you experience any fear, anxiety or tension during the birth? Mother: Father:

6. How did the physical pain (or pleasure) of your DIY compare to other births?

7. Was your length of labor shorter than other births? Estimate the length of labor for each child:

PART IV. BIRTH STORY

I am interested in your detailed stories about "DIY" children born after 1/1/90. You may make reference to other births, but the real focus should be on those after 1/1/90.   If you have had more than one DIY since 1/1/90, I would be interested in knowing what you did differently from one birth to the next.

Now it is time for you to tell your story. At this time, I have no length restrictions. You may attach your story to the rest of this questionnaire. In many cases, the mother has written about the couple's experience. Please indicate who is writing the story. In this project, however, in order for your work to be included in my book, *I must have at least one written page from fathers. (O.K., the mother can write it down, but it must be a transcript of what the father is saying.) I want to know how the homebirth changed the man's life, how he felt about everything. I want you to bear your soul, father.* A major part of my book depends upon the male experience.

PART V. CONCLUDING THOUGHTS

1. Did you have the birth videotaped, photographed, audiotaped? What were the pros and cons in your experience?

2. What would you like to do differently next time regarding the pregnancy or actual birth?

3. Give me a few adjectives to describe 3 months postpartum following your homebirth. If the birth story you wrote about was not your 1st child, how does this postpartum period compare with earlier birth experiences?

4. How has the DIY changed both (the mother and father) of your lives? Do you feel more connected to your mate, your child?

5. If you have had a DIY homebirth and would not do a DIY again, why?

6. Bibliography or a few resources that were invaluable to you in your preparation for a homebirth.

7. Is there anything else you want to tell me? Any other suggestions or comments?

8. What topics should be written about / researched regarding homebirths?

PART VI.   FOR PARENTS WHO HAVE HAD THEIR FIRST BABY A DIY HOMEBIRTH

1. When did you decide to have an unassisted homebirth?

2. How did you know to have a DIY homebirth? Where did you learn about DIY homebirths?

GLOSSARY

abruptio placenta accidental hemorrhage. The peeling away of part of the placenta from the wall of the uterus in late pregnancy, which may result in heavy bleeding.

alphafetoprotein (AFP) a substance produced by the embryonic yolk sac, and later by the fetal liver, which enters the mother's bloodstream during pregnancy. A very high level can indicate neural tube defects of the fetus—such as Down's syndrome or spina bifida—but can also mean a multiple pregnancy.

amniotomy the surgical rupture of the amniotic sac, sometimes done to speed up labor. Also referred to as ARM (artificial rupture of the membranes).

blood pressure (BP) pressure extended by the blood upon the walls of the blood vessels, (especially arteries) and usually measured on the radial artery.

cephalopelvic disproportion (CPD) a state in which the head of the baby is assumed to be larger than the cavity of the mother's pelvis. Delivery must be by C-section.

certified nurse midwife (CNM) a graduate of an approved program who is licensed to practice by her state

cesarean section (C-section) delivery of the baby through a cut in the abdominal and uterine walls.

chorionic villus sampling (CVS) a tiny sample of tissue is taken from the chorionic villi, which are fingerlike projections of tissue that surround the baby in the early weeks and ultimately form the placenta. CVS can be performed between 8-11 weeks gestation.

dilatation and curettage (D & C) the surgical opening of the cervix and removal of the contents of the uterus.

do-it-yourself (DIY) term used to describe actions performed in the absence of trained, skilled, or paid professionals.

doula labor assistant; Greek term meaning "in service of."

dystocia, shoulder a state in which the baby's shoulders get stuck during delivery.

electronic fetal monitor (EFM) instrument used to monitor the fetal heart rate during labor. A transducer is placed on the abdomen over the area of the fetal heart (external) or an electrode is inserted throught the cervix and clipped to the baby's scalp (internal).

epidural regional anesthesia, used during labor in which an anesthetic is injected through a catheter into the epidural space in the lower spine.

episiotomy a surgical cut in the perineum to enlarge the vagina.

hematocrit an instrument for determining the relative amounts of plasma and corpuscles in the blood.

homeschooling home-based educational approach involving parents and their children.

iatrogenic doctor-caused.

intensive care unit (ICU) special medical facilities, services, and monitoring devices to meet the needs of gravely ill patients.

intravenous drip (IV) the infusion offluids directly into the bloodstream by means of a fine catheter introduced into a vein.

Kegel exercise done to tighten the perineal muscles.

meconium the first contents of the bowel, present in the fetus before birth and passed during the first days after birth. The presence of meconium in the fluid before delivery is usually viewed as a sign of fetal distress.

monitrice labor assistant; French term meaning "a woman who watches over attentively."

natural family planning (NFP) fertility awareness method in which the goal is to avoid or achieve pregnancy through a combination of observing cervical mucus, condition of the cervix, and basal temperature.

oxytocin hormone secreted by the pituitary gland which

stimulates uterine contractions and the milk glands in the breasts to produce milk.

perineal message also perineum message. Exercising and stretching of the skin and tissues around the vaginal opening.

Phenylketonuria (PKU) an extremely rare metabolic disorder occuring in approximately 1 out of 15,000 infants. If diagnosed shortly after birth, it can often be treated with a special diet, but if left untreated, it can result in brain damage.

pitocin syntheitc form of oxytocin, often used to induce or accelerate labor. It is sometimes used to stop bleeding.

placenta previa a condition where the placenta lies over the cervix. It can result in hemorrhage. Cesarean sections are performed in cases of complete placenta previa.

placental abruption (abruptio placenta) all or part of the placenta separates from the uterine wall.

postpartum after delivery.

prolapsed cord umbilical cord comes through the birth canal in advance of the baby.

Reiki Japanese word representing Universal Life Energy, the energy which is all around us. It is derived from *rei*, meaning "transcendental spirit, or "universal" and *ki*, meaning "vital life force energy." System of healing that utilizes specific techniques for restoring and balancing the natural life force energy within the body. It is a holistic, natural and hands-on system that affects the mind, body and spirit.

Rhesus factor a distinguishing characteristic of the red blood corpuscles. Human beings have either Rhesus positive or Rhesus negative blood. If the mother is Rhesus negative and the fetus Rhesus positive severe complications and Rhesus disease (the destruction of the red corpuscles by antibodies) may occur.

supine position back-laying position commonly used in hospital deliveries.

ultrasound also referred to as sonogram. A method of producing a picture of an object by bouncing high frequency sound waves off of it. Ultrasound is used to show the development of the fetus in the uterus.

unassisted birth after cesearean(UBAC) term which indicates an unassisted birth after a previous C-section.

unassisted homebirth giving birth without a doctor or midwife, commonly occuring at home. Also referred to as unassisted birth, unassisted childbirth, do-it-yourself birth, freebirth, unattended birth.

unschooling an approach to homeschooling that is unstructured and child-centered. Also referred to as self-directed learning.

vaginal birth after cesearean (VBAC) term coined by Nancy Wainer Cohen in 1974 to indicate a vaginal birth after a previous C-section.

BIBLIOGRAPHY

Arms, Suzanne. *Immaculate Deception: A New Look at Women and Childbirth in America.* 1975, Houghton Mifflin, Co., Boston, MA.

Armstrong, Penny, C.N.M. and Feldman, Sheryl. *A Wise Birth: Bringing Together the Best of Natural Childbirth With Modern Medicine.* 1990, William Morrow & Co., Inc., NY.

Baker, Jeannine Parvati. *Prenatal Yoga and Natural Birth.* 1986, Freestone Innerprizes, P.O. Box 398, Monroe, UT 84754

_____. "The Possible Family: Little House on the Edge of the Millennium." 1995, Freestone Innerprizes, Monroe, UT.

_____. "The Shamanic Dimensions of Childbirth." Freestone Innerprizes, Monroe, UT.

_____. "Shamanic Midwifery: Hands that Heal Birth." Freestone Innerprizes, Monroe, UT.

Baldwin, Rahima. *Special Delivery.* 1986, Celestial Arts, Berkeley, CA.

Balizet, Carol. *Born in Zion: A Journal of True Adventures in Learning the Faithfulness of God.* 1992, Christ Center Publishing International, Euless, TX.

Beckelman, Laurie. *Grief.* 1995, Crestwood House, Parsippany, NJ.

Benson, Michael D., M.D. *Birth Day! The Last 24 Hours of Pregnancy.* 1993, Paragon House, NY, NY.

Brackhill, Yvonne, Rice, June and Young, Diony. *Birth Trap: How to Avoid the Dangers of High-tech Hospital*

Delivery-and Where to Find Alternatives. 1984, Warner Books, NY, NY.

Carter, Patricia Cloyd. *Come Gently, Sweet Lucina.* 1957, Patricia Cloyd Carter, Titusville, FL.

Cain, Kathy. *Partners in Birth: Your Complete Guide to Helping a Mother Give Birth.* 1990, Warner Books, NY, NY.

Corsini, Raymond J., ed. *Encyclopedia of Psychology, Vol. 2.* 1984. John E. Wiley & Sons, NY. p. 161.

Davis-Floyd, Robbie. "Hospital Birth as a Technocratic Rite of Passage." *Mothering,* Summer 1993, pp. 69-74.

Del Mazza, Valentino. *Secrets for Finding Happiness in Marriage.* 1984, Daughters of St. Paul, Boston, MA.

Dick-Read, Grantly, M. D. *Childbirth Without Fear: The Principles and Practice of Natural Childbirth,* 2nd Ed. 1959, Harper & Row Publishers, NY.

Friedan, Betty. *The Second Stage.* 1981, Summit Books, NY, NY.

Gaskin, Ina May. *Spiritual Midwifery,* 3rd Ed. 1990, The Book Publishing Co., Summertown, TN.

Gilgoff, Alice. *Home Birth: An Invitation and a Guide.* 1989, Bergin & Garvey Publishers, Inc., MA.

Estes, Clarissa Pinkola, PhD. *Women Who Run With the Wolves: Myths and Stories of the Wild Woman Archetype.* 1992, Ballentine Books, NY.

Hazell, Lester Dassez. *Commonsense Childbirth.* 1976, G. P. Putnam's Sons, NY, NY.

Henry, Sherrye. *The Deep Divide: Why American Women Resist Equality.* 1994, Macmillan Pub., Co., NY, NY.

Imbiorski, Walter J. & Thomas, John L., *Beginning Your Marriage.* 1969, Delaney Pub., Chicago, Ill.

Jones, Carl. *Mind Over Labor: How to Reduce the Fear and Pain of Childbirth through Mental Imagery.* 1987, Viking Penguin, Inc., NY, NY.

_____. *Visualizations for an Easier Childbirth.* 1988, Meadowbrook, Simon & Schuster, NY, NY.

Kitzinger, Sheila. *Homebirth: The Essential Guide to*

Giving Birth Outside of the Hospital. 1991, Dorling Kindersley, Inc., NY, NY.

Korte, Diana and Scaer, Roberta. *A Good Birth, A Safe Birth.* 1990, Bantam, NY, NY.

Kübler-Ross, Elisabeth. *On Death and Dying.* 1969, The Macmillan Co., Inc., NY, NY.

Leboyer, Frederick. *Birth Without Violence.* 1975, Alfred A. Knopf, Inc., Random House, NY.

LeShan, Eda J. *The Conspiracy Against Childhood.* 1968, McClelland & Stewart Ltd., H. Wolff, NY.

Louv, Richard. *Childhood's Future: Listening to the American Family. New Hope for the Next Generation.* 1990, Houghton Mifflin, Co., MA.

Macfarlane, Aidan. *The Psychology of Childbirth.* 1977, Harvard University Press, Cambridge, MA.

Mann, Judy. *The Difference: Growing Up Female in America.* 1994, Warner Books, Inc., NY, NY.

Maslow, Abraham H. *Toward a Psychology of Being,* 2nd ed. 1968, Van Nostrand Reinhold Co., NY, NY.

McCutcheon-Rosegg, Susan and Rosegg, Peter. *Natural Childbirth the Bradley Way.* 1984, Plume/Penguin Books.

Mendelsohn, Robert, M.D. *How to Raise a Healthy Child in Spite of Your Doctor.* 1984, Ballantine Books, NY.

_____. *Male Practice: How Doctors Manipulate Women.* 1982, Contemporary Books, Inc., Chicago, Ill.

Mother Teresa of Calcutta. *Gift for God: Prayers and Meditations.* 1975, Harper & Row, Publishers, NY, NY.

Moran, Marilyn A. *Birth and the Dialogue of Love.* 1981, New Nativity Press, Reading, MA.

_____ed. *Happy Birth Days: Personal Accounts of Birth at Home the Intimate, Husband / Wife Way.* 1986, New Nativity Press, Reading, MA.

_____. *Pleasurable Husband/Wife Childbirth: The Real Consummation of Married Love.* 1997, New Nativity Press, Reading, MA.

Napierala, Susanna. *Water Birth: A Midwife's Perspective.*

1994, Bergin & Garvey, Westport, CT.

Odent, Michel. *Birth Reborn: How Childbirth Can Be What Women Want it to be—and How Mothers and Babies Both Benefit.* 1984, Random House, NY.

_____. *The Nature of Birth and Breastfeeding.* 1992, Bergin & Garvey, Westport, CT.

Perez, Polly. "Someone to Watch Over Her: Professional Labor Support," *Childbirth Instructor,* Autumn 1993, pp. 22-26.

Pride, Mary. *All the Way Home: Power for Your Family to be its Best.* 1989, Crossway Books, Wheaton, Ill.

_____. *The Way Home: Beyond Feminism, Back to Reality.* 1985. Crossway Books, Wheaton, Ill.

Rothman, Barbara Katz. *In Labor: Women and Power in the Birthplace.* 1982, W.W. Norton & Co., NY, NY.

Ryckman, Richard M. *Theories of Personality*, 2nd Ed. 1982, Brooks / Cole Publishing Co., Monterey, CA.

Sears, Martha, R.N. & William, M.D. *The Birth Book: Everything You Need to Know to Have a Safe and Satisfying Birth.* 1994, Little, Brown & Co., Boston, MA.

Shanley, Laura Kaplan. *Unassisted Childbirth.* 1994, Bergin & Garvey, Westport, CT.

Sheen, Fulton J. *Love, Marriage and Children.* 1954, Dell Pub. Co., Inc., NY, NY.

Sommers, Christina Hoff. *Who Stole Feminism? How Women have Betrayed Women.* 1994, Simon & Schuster, NY, NY.

Sousa, Marion. *Childbirth at Home.* 1976, Prentice-Hall Inc., Englewood Cliffs, NJ.

St. Paul Editions. *The Love Covenant.* 1983, Daughters of St. Paul, Boston, MA.

Stewart, David, PhD. *The Five Standards for Safe Childbearing.* 1981 (1st Ed.) and 1997 (2nd Ed.), NAPSAC International, Marble Hill, MO.

Walton, Vicki. *Have it Your Way.* 1976, Henry Phillips Publishing Co., NY.

White, Gregory, M.D. *Emergency Childbirth: A Manaual.* 1989, Police Training Foundation, Franklin Park, Ill.

Wolf, Naomi. *The Beauty Myth: How Images of Beauty are Used Against Women.* 1991, William & Morrow Pub., Co. NY.

⎯⎯⎯⎯⎯. *Fire with Fire: The New Female Power and How it will Change the 21ˢᵗ Century.* 1993, Random House, NY.

Young, Catherine. *Mother's Best Secrets.* 1992, Mother Press, Ontario, Canada.

Index